Read
Yourself
Happy

Read Yourself *Happy*

How to use books to ease your anxiety

DAISY BUCHANAN

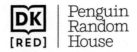

First published in Great Britain in 2025 by
DK RED, an imprint of
Dorling Kindersley Limited
20 Vauxhall Bridge Road,
London SW1V 2SA

The authorised representative in the EEA is
Dorling Kindersley Verlag GmbH. Arnulfstr. 124,
80636 Munich, Germany

A CIP catalogue record for this book
is available from the British Library.
HB ISBN: 978-0-2416-9165-6

Printed and bound in the United Kingdom

www.dk.com

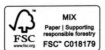

MIX
Paper | Supporting
responsible forestry
FSC™ C018179

This book was made with Forest
Stewardship Council™ certified
paper – one small step in DK's
commitment to a sustainable future.
Learn more at **www.dk.com/uk/
information/sustainability**

For readers and worriers everywhere

Contents

Introduction

Dear reader, how are you feeling right now? Really. I hope you're sitting somewhere comfortable and quiet. I hope you're feeling calm, still, and unhurried. I hope your heartbeat is steady and your breath is even. I hope you're here.

But I understand that's an awful lot to hope for.

You might instead be reading this on the bus, sitting in traffic, and trying to fight the rising feeling of panic and anxiety as you calculate how late you're going to be. You might be reading this in the bathroom because it's the one place you can go where your kids will give you five minutes' peace (or maybe just two or three). Perhaps you're reading because you can't sleep, trying to distract yourself from the list of unfinished tasks that keeps circulating in your head. We all have so much on our minds that simply stopping to read might cause your anxiety to spike rather than calm you.

My asking might be the first time today that you've had a chance to think about how you're feeling. Now you're checking in with your body, you may be surprised to discover that the anxiety seems to be sitting in your jaw or there's tension in your toes.

Many of us are struggling. We've been struggling for a while. The world is full of things to react to and worry about – and sometimes managing our anxiety seems like another exhausting task to add to the list. I have generalised anxiety disorder (GAD), which has made me feel frightened, isolated, and lonely. When my anxiety has been at its worst, it has made me feel like I'm the only person in the world who can't cope. Yet, ironically, I am not alone – anxiety has never been more widespread. According to mental health charity Mind, in England, six in every 100 people are diagnosed with GAD every week,[1] and Mental Health UK reports that, in the UK, eight million people are experiencing an anxiety disorder of some kind at any one time.[2]

The first thing I'd like to tell you is that you're not alone either, you're part of a gang. Here, you don't have to worry about worrying. It's fine to let yourself be anxious, if that's the way you're feeling right now. Anxiety works like an oversensitive smoke alarm: it's hyper-responsive and it's trying to keep us safe. We don't feel this way because something has gone wrong, and we don't feel this way because something is wrong with us. I wish I could switch your brain off for a while, but I can't. What I can do, though, is tell you that you're safe here, in this moment, and I'm with you. What I won't do is tell you about cannabidiol (CBD) oil, the benefits of regular exercise, long, hot baths, or ask you if you've tried mindfulness. (In the spirit of full disclosure, I've found all these things to be useful and enjoyable. However, when I've been on the floor, figuratively and literally, I could have punched anyone who suggested that I could be fixed by taking a bath.)

I would also like to tell you about an anxiety-easing habit that I believe in with my whole heart. Ever since I was little – long before I understood what anxiety was or why I had it – I've instinctively practised this habit and used it to self-soothe. You're doing it right now.

When I'm feeling anxious, I read. Reading makes me feel calm, curious, and connected. Stories hold me, absorb me, and deliver the stillness I am seeking. And – I can't stress this enough – I am not Ron Burgundy, and I do not have many leather-bound books. If I'm feeling deeply anxious, I don't pick up the sort of book I might want to show off about at a dinner party. I'm looking instead for old friends, stories I might already be familiar with. Soft places to land. We're talking Sweet Valley High, The Princess Diaries and The Baby-sitters' Club series of books. I know *Bridget Jones's Diary* almost off by heart because I've been turning to it since I was a teenager.

You, too, can read any book you like. You'll know what your comfort stories are. Maybe you take refuge in a Mick Herron, crave an Adrian Mole, Spot the Dog, or *The Unbearable Lightness of Being* (hey, I'm not fancy, but you might be!). Whatever you choose, I'd love to show you – or perhaps remind you – that reading isn't a chore. It's not an adult homework task or another overwhelming activity to add to your enormous list. It's a happy habit, and it's just for you. No one needs to know what you're reading, when you're reading, and how much you're reading. The important thing, I strongly believe, is that, if you can find a tiny bit of time to read, you'll be finding a way to ease your anxiety. With a book, you can be completely present in your body, while escaping the world for a bit. Sometimes it takes me a little time to find the silence, but I keep reading and it turns the volume down on the increasingly hectic world around us.

Before we get started, I'd like to make one thing very clear. It's important that you don't feel guilty or ashamed about not reading 'enough' or reading the 'wrong' sort of book. Most of all, I want to make the case for reading in a way that works for you, and I explore why so many of us *do* feel bad about what we read and how much we read. During my most anxious periods, I've picked up serious books, searching for solace, and sometimes those books have left me confused and alienated. When a painful experience at work left me feeling burned out and broken, I tried to read *How to Be Both* by Ali Smith, which had just won the Women's Prize for Fiction.

It did not go well.

I remember sitting on a train and feeling the weight of the book in my lap and the weight of my phone in my hand. Trying to read a sentence, I was skidding over the words too quickly, unable to find purchase or process their meaning. It was as though my mental tyre treads were completely worn out and I couldn't grip on to anything to direct my thoughts and get where I wanted to go. I'd look at the book, then blink, and realise that I was looking at my phone. Then I'd look out of the window and wonder what was wrong with me. Then I'd look at my phone again. It was no wonder that I felt so scared at work and so bad at my job. I was so useless that I couldn't even read the first page of an important, prize-winning novel!

I felt sad and stupid. Reading had always been there for me.

When I was being bullied at primary school, I turned to books to make me feel happy and safe. As a teenager struggling to navigate the world, books made me feel hopeful. In sleepy, conservative, rural Dorset, I sat in the library and fell in love with Tennessee Williams and George Orwell. I dreamed of cities, parties, and revolutions. During lonely moments at university, I cheered myself up with old friends from home – Marian Keyes, Truman Capote, Armistead Maupin. Books had always been good to me. They had offered me safety and escape, comfort, joy, *and* adventure. All they'd ever asked from me was my attention and now I couldn't even give this one that.

At the time, I didn't realise that I was badly burned out. I was furious with myself for being unable to switch off, concentrate, or get into a flow state. Back then, I didn't think of myself as a human being, having human responses to some relatively new stimulus. I had a love–hate relationship with social media and my smartphone. I felt 'addicted' and I was angry about being unable to control myself. It did not occur to me that I felt addicted because it had been designed to be addictive.

When I'm describing a book I love, I often find myself falling back on the old cliché 'I couldn't put it down.' When I say this, it's true – the experience of being immersed in the story is so powerful that I don't want to be anywhere else. With a book, this experience has only ever made me feel good – connected, exhilarated, and present. Yet, my phone is the ultimate 'I couldn't put it down' read. I pick up my phone when I want to feel connected, but it has never made me feel exhilarated or present. It has made me feel overwhelmed, lonely, scattered, and exhausted.

Don't worry – I'm not asking you to give up your phone. I am asking you to give yourself a bit of grace and generosity when it comes to understanding your existing habits and how they might be exacerbating your anxiety. Here is what I wish I'd known, back then. My reading habit is a muscle and, just like a physical muscle, I need to use it regularly to keep it strong. Also just like a physical muscle, I needed to build it up slowly. On the train, I'd attempted the book version of going to a brand-new gym and picking up the heaviest weight, with no training or guidance.

Of course I dropped the weight, hurt my back, and felt sulky and unfit. I needed to work out very gently for just a few minutes every day. I needed to start with some smaller weights and let myself remember the way that they felt. Perhaps you can consider this book your set of training weights as you come with me, exploring a wide range of subjects, themes, and genres together, and the books that will help us to navigate our biggest, smallest, and most confusing emotions. As your page-turning personal trainer, I promise not to push you into anything before you feel ready. I hope, working together, you will achieve the results you want – a reading habit that brings you happiness and joy, one that makes you feel so good, you don't care what anyone else thinks about it.

After struggling with *How to Be Both,* I returned to a childhood favourite, one of The Baby-sitters' Club books. I read for comfort and for calm. I discovered that a beloved book can be like a favourite sweater, and all that matters is it makes you feel soft and warm. I needed to heal and spend time repairing my relationship with reading before I was ready to move on.

Some years later, I opened *How to Be Both* and tried again. I felt anxious and trepidatious but, this time, every sentence drew me closer to the story. The book captured my attention and held it. I felt myself relaxing into its universe and I felt confident and connected. I had been training regularly. My strength had been increasing, slowly and imperceptibly. As I read, 'I fell in love the way you fall asleep: slowly, and then all at once.'[3] At last, I was ready for the giant literary dumb-bell.

If you've ever lost yourself in a story, this book is for you. It's a celebration of books and reading – and it's an invitation to reconnect with an instinctive, human part of yourself. We have been sharing, telling, and listening to stories since before we even had written language. We are all descended from generations of story lovers.

This book is also for anyone who just feels lost. If that's you, I believe you can find yourself in a story. Maybe it's been a while since you loved a book so much that you couldn't put it down because switching off is such a struggle. I want to help you to find the right book. I promise, it's a passport that will let you take a holiday from your own head. If you reconnect with reading, you can bring some order to your thoughts and ease that seemingly endless feeling of dread.

I spend a lot of time speaking with readers and asking them why they keep turning to certain books. Some of you might listen to the podcast I host, You're Booked, in which I interview my favourite authors (and yours!) about the stories that have formed them and the books they keep coming back to. As well as reading stories, I write them. I'm the author of four novels – *Insatiable, Careering, Limelight,* **and** *Pity Party.* I write because I read. I'm interested in talking with writers who read, too, because they care about the way books make them feel. Throughout this book, I'll be including interviews with experts and authors about how books soothe, move, challenge, and captivate us. I've discovered that reading is a club *anyone* is welcome to join. As readers, all of us can rub shoulders with icons and legends.

Reading is so good for us, but possibly not in the way that we have been led to believe. Yes, reading can increase our knowledge, fuel our curiosity, and strengthen our empathy. Books also allow us to travel all over the world and can teach us history, philosophy, and geography. But, in all honesty, those aren't the lessons I remember. The most lasting thing I've learned from reading is that we're never alone. First, it doesn't matter how mad, sad, or obscure our dilemma is, someone else has lived it and written down everything they discovered and everything they felt. Second, during those moments when our feelings are overwhelming and difficult to bear, a book is the most generous friend we could hope to find. A book meets us where we are, absorbing our sadness and distracting us from it. When my anxiety overwhelms me, I feel very scared of uncertainty and unable to deal with the unknown. But the best books encourage me to embrace uncertainty. I want to read a story because I don't know what's going to happen or how it will end. The more I enjoy the uncertainty of stories, the better I get at tolerating uncertainty in life.

We've all been forced to muddle our way through a book that didn't excite us or engage us. How would you feel if you had permission to read anything? And, just as important, you don't have to read everything! You're allowed to try whatever you like the look of and don't have to justify that choice to anyone. You can read any book in the *Sunday Times* review section, any book you discover on TikTok, or any book you find on the shelves of your local charity shop. It doesn't matter where your books come from, I believe the act of reading will always leave you feeling better than when it found you.

Together, we're going on a grand tour. We'll be exploring how books can bring us comfort and support when we're at our lowest, and how reading can ease the physical and mental symptoms of intense stress. We'll look at how books can help us to make sense of our complicated families. We'll discover how books can enhance our lives, increase our capacity for joy, and make us feel more connected to the people we love. We'll find out how books can make us funnier, braver – and hornier. We'll even learn how reading can help us to find meaning and purpose when global events make us feel powerless. At the end of every chapter, I'll be sharing some book recommendations, and the aim of this is to bring you inspiration, comfort, and joy. Maybe you'll spot some of your own old favourites among them, but I also hope to introduce you to some brand-new books that you will love.

When we're in anxiety's grip, it can feel impossible to ask for the help that we desperately need. We can't explain ourselves. We can't make ourselves heard. I wish I could cure our anxiety and make sure that we all feel safe, happy, and confident for ever. I can't do that, but I can do the next best thing. I can share everything I know about the habit that has soothed and restored me, helping me to forge a path through my darkest moments.

Come with me and I'll show you how reading has eased my anxiety and can ease yours too. I promise, there is a book out there that will fill your heart and blow your mind. If you're feeling anxious and isolated, reading will make you feel connected. It's the best medicine I know.

1

Read yourself CALMER

"The yawn marked the end of a mood of anxiety"

Henry Williamson [1]

I'm only eight years old, but I have a *lot* on. Mentally, I've got a packed schedule. School is first on the list, as it's the place where most things go wrong.

Staying near the top of the class, being quiet, being good, and keeping my teachers happy – that's relatively easy, although I often get told off for my terrible handwriting. Avoiding the mean girls and bullies is a lot harder.

I've been told to 'ignore' them. On the radio, I hear a news story about someone who died because they slept through an earthquake and suspect that they were probably very good at ignoring bullies. I'm not.

And now, I need to add earthquakes to my list of concerns. My parents reassure me that, in the UK, they're *rare*. 'Rare' does not reassure me. 'Rare' does not mean 'it has never happened and it never will happen'. I will probably die in an earthquake, if I don't get poisoned first. Mum keeps bleach and sprays in the kitchen cupboard under the sink and every time I close my eyes, I see the skull and crossbones logo on the label. I'd never be so stupid as to touch the bleach, but what if I ate some by accident?

At night, I lie awake, listing the times I may have accidentally ingested bleach. Just the other day, one of my sisters was sick on the carpet. Mum has definitely used something scary to clean it up. What if I touched it without realising? I'm probably dying right now. I can feel the heat rising in my cheeks and my heart is pounding. I'll be gone by morning. Crying quietly, I wait to die.

But at 6am, I'm still alive. I leap out of bed and ask my mother what specifically she used for cleaning up the sick and whether it's poisonous.

She thinks for a moment. 'Dettol,' she replies at last. I'm reassured. We've had lots of conversations about Dettol. I know it's a household disinfectant spray, and the tiny quantity that will have been sprayed on the carpet isn't strong enough to poison me.

But then I remember, there was a subsequent carpet-cleaning episode, with spilled milk. Maybe there was something else used for that and it's about to take effect. 'And when Grace knocked over her mug last night, what did you use then?'

'Ditto.'

In a faltering voice, I ask, 'Is Ditto poisonous?'

Worrying about worrying

I have always been a worrier. I worried my way through school, exams, university, job interviews, and hangovers. I assumed I was simply wired that way – my father and sisters worried too. My mother seemed more laid back, but she'd often say things like, 'Well, does it really matter when we'll all be dead one day?' At the time, that didn't help at all. When I went to an all-girls grammar school, worry seemed to be in the water. I look back at that time and I don't know whether I want to laugh or shake Past Me and my friends.

On any given day, we'd ruminate obsessively on the following: the war in Iraq, the likelihood of failing all our exams and becoming completely unemployable, our impending student debt, the likelihood of never falling in love and dying alone, the state of our skin, our hatred of our bodies, and the tragic death of Princess Diana. My friendship group was obsessed with the film *Titanic* – ostensibly because we all loved Leonardo DiCaprio, but I suspect it was really because there was something oddly reassuring about exposing ourselves to tragedy and disaster. We all feared the worst. Somehow it helped to go to the cinema and watch the worst.

I worried, I worried about my worrying, and I did my very best to distract myself from the worry. Food helped – that was my first love, my first drug, and an effective way to feel numb, quickly. In my teens, I added alcohol to my arsenal and, in my 20s, I found that shopping worked, too, for a little while. Of course, drugs wear off, and my worry always came roaring back. It was just an unfortunate part of my personality and I had to learn to live with it – or at least hide from it, crush it, and try to pretend it didn't exist, until it felt so overwhelming and terrifying that I couldn't feel anything else.

The first time I heard the term 'generalised anxiety disorder' (GAD for short), I was 24 and in my GP's surgery. I'd made the appointment because I hurt my back, but when the doctor asked me how I was in general, I burst into tears. When he wrote me a prescription for antidepressants (citalopram), I wept again, but with joy and relief. I didn't have to be 'a worrier'. I was *ill*, which meant that, one day, I might feel better.

The pills didn't cure me. My anxiety would get better, then worse. But my diagnosis made me feel seen and heard for the very first time. Memories that had been fogged by relentless stress and worry suddenly appeared in sharp focus. I didn't want to feel the way I always felt, and maybe I didn't have to. Maybe there was a way to feel better.

The age of anxiety

When I first saw my doctor, I didn't know anyone else who had been diagnosed with GAD. Now, 15 years later, I'd struggle to name a friend who *hasn't* been diagnosed with it. In 2023, the Mental Health Foundation found that 73 per cent of people had struggled with anxiety sometimes in the previous two weeks, and 20 per cent of people had felt anxious 'most or all of the time'.[2] The charity Mental Health UK estimates that as many as eight million people in the UK could be living with an anxiety disorder.[3] It's difficult to be precise about numbers because so many people aren't able to access the mental health support they need.

It's important to point out that anxiety is a very common, very human emotional state. Everyone feels anxious sometimes. We all worry about the world we live in and the details of our lives. Anxiety might be the one thing we all have in common. It doesn't matter what your circumstances are, no one can completely avoid having concerns about family, work, relationships, money, housing, and health.

We could be forgiven for thinking that the 21st century is a more anxious one than previous centuries, especially in the aftermath of the Covid pandemic and seismic political upheavals that have happened. But we've been talking about – and worrying about – all kinds of things for thousands of years. Clinical researcher and anxiety specialist Marc-Antoine Crocq writes that Cicero 'makes an interesting distinction between *anxietas* that designates trait anxiety or the fact of being prone to [general] anxiousness, and *angor* that refers to state anxiety or current anxiety'.[4] In fact, Cicero's ancient writing argues that our mental state has a physical impact on us – a concept that felt new in 2014 when Bessel van der Kolk published his book on the subject, *The Body Keeps the Score*. We can't even claim that we live in some new 'age of anxiety' as this phrase was coined by W. H. Auden, whose poem of the same name won the Pulitzer Prize in 1948.

When you feel overwhelmed by anxiety, I hope it helps to remember that it doesn't mean something is wrong with you. Your brain and body are responding to the world in a very human way. Indeed, humans have been feeling anxious – and trying to ease that feeling – since records began.

However, we are living through an especially overwhelming era. When Cicero was observing and documenting anxiety, he was doing so at a time before rolling newsfeeds, smartphones, and relentless cycles of information. At the time of writing, the headlines are dominated by war in Ukraine and Gaza. The news isn't confined to newspapers or even TV, we're bombarded by violent and devastating images everywhere we go. Psychology professor Alison Holman studied a group of people who watched six hours or more of news every day for a week after the Boston Marathon bombings in 2013. She found that these people suffered more from acute stress than those who had lost loved ones or seen the explosion in person. 'I think people really strongly, deeply underestimate the impact the news can have,' she told the BBC.[5]

Rolf Dobelli, author of *The Art of Thinking Clearly,* wrote in an essay about the effects of news on us, 'news is to the mind what sugar is to the body... News is toxic to your body. It constantly triggers the limbic system. Panicky stories spur the release of cascades of glucocorticoid (cortisol). This deregulates your immune system and inhibits the release of growth hormones. In other words, your body finds itself in a state of chronic stress.'[6]

Jill Hanney, a psychotherapist and trauma specialist, told me that, among her patients, she noticed panic attacks went up in the period following the start of the Covid pandemic in 2020. She suspects that the rolling news cycle contributed to our collective anxiety. 'If horror is coming into your living room night after night,' she says, 'your brain experiences it as stress. Our brains are incredibly complex and clever, but on some levels they can't tell the difference between something happening on a screen in front of us and something that is actually happening to us. We produce more adrenaline and cortisol, and have core reactions, as though we're experiencing what we're seeing.'

Scroll survivors

As well as the serious stuff, there's the local news – and our hyperlocal news. If you're an Instagram user, and you pull out your phone and scroll when you're bored at work or waiting in a supermarket queue, you might be presented with a lot of potentially emotive information. You might see posts about violent crime and global disaster. You might learn that someone you went to school with is pregnant – neutral news that feels anything but neutral if you're trying for a baby yourself. You might see an ad claiming some big celebrity swears by a particular mascara and find yourself buying it before you have had a chance to draw breath.

I was anxious long before I had a smartphone, but I have no doubt that it exacerbates my anxiety. When I use it, I'm continually reading and digesting information, but I'm in a reactive state. Sometimes it makes me feel as though I've lost custody of my thoughts and emotions. My phone regularly presents me with unsolicited information that makes me feel scared, angry, sad, or envious. Then it tells me that I might feel better if I bought something, a process it's quick to facilitate.

Considering the way that we consume news and information might hold the key to understanding our anxious tendencies. Our anxious brains are desperate for information. We believe that the more we can learn about a subject, the better we can plan and prepare for it. The problem is that the information seems infinite and it's available to us instantly.

Becca Caddy, author of *Screen Time: How to make peace with your devices and find techquilibrium,* explains, 'Many of us reach for our phones because it takes less effort to passively scroll than it does to actively engage in an activity or hobby. There's a time and a place for passive scrolling, but too much of it can leave us feeling drained and unfulfilled and frustrated with our lack of willpower. It's that frustration which I think is a big problem for a lot of us.'

I'm reassured when she tells me, 'We're layering extra pressure and panic on when we judge ourselves for reaching for our phones. After all, they're designed to be shiny, colourful, filled with notifications, and other virtual treats. They're designed to make us want to reach for them over and over.'

She explains that we're all different and we all respond to these stimuli differently. 'For some people, restrictions can help. I often put my phone in do not disturb mode or airplane mode when I have lots to do. Others don't do well when further demands are placed on them and it can lead to even more procrastination and judgement. These people might actually find unlimited screen time and zero judgement ends up helping them in the long run. Or assigning certain times of the day when you're allowed to scroll.'

It's reassuring to know that there's not necessarily one right way to handle the challenges of this kind of hyper-connection. We just need to work out what is right for us and pay attention to the way we feel in our bodies. It's taken me a long time and a lot of practice to learn to do this. In her Substack newsletter, 'How to Survive an Existential Crisis', poet Nikita Gill wrote, 'The urge to scroll can be replaced as any habit can. I taught myself to keep a book by my phone and when I am about to grab my phone, I go for the book now. I keep reminding myself that it is better to read a page of a good book than learn why GaryMcGuy83746421 thinks women aren't actual people.'[7] Like Nikita, I've realised that, while habits are hard to disrupt, we have the power to stop, think, and change. Over time, I've noticed that I tend to reach for my phone when I want to feel soothed and connected, even though it almost always delivers information that makes me feel overwhelmed and dysregulated. A book doesn't bring me the same instant, fizzy hit of distraction but, when I force myself to focus on the page, I eventually find the soothing sensation I crave. The effects take longer to kick in, but they last a lot longer.

Anxiety and the pandemic

Many of my most anxious friends told me that their relationship with anxiety started to change in the spring of 2020. 'Most of my anxiety is connected to a fear of losing control,' says Maria, a 30-year-old HR manager. 'I worry obsessively about missing appointments and deadlines, that everything will go horribly wrong, *and it will all be my fault*. Of course, when lockdown was announced, there was a reason to be anxious. It affected everyone, people were dying or getting seriously ill. We all had to put our lives on hold. But my anxiety itself became much easier to bear because I knew my response was a proportionate one. I worried, but the physical symptoms lessened. And the light started to get in. It gave me the mental space to look for things to ease that anxiety.'

Like Maria, I was surprised – and a little guilty – to discover that managing my mental health felt a tiny bit easier during the pandemic. I worried obsessively over the things I could control, but I had no control at all over this global disaster. And I noticed that the news had a significant, measurable impact on my anxiety. Well, I noticed that there was no news. It was possible to devote whole days to reading about Covid, the predicted length of lockdown, and what the government was going to do, but I wasn't really learning anything. It wasn't helping.

But my brain wanted something to digest. I craved information. And I was a reader. I loved books. I hosted a books podcast. I usually had at least one novel on the go, but I wasn't prioritising my reading habit – I could usually find time for it, but I wasn't going out of my way to *make* time for it. At that point, plenty of people were making noises about using lockdown for self-improvement projects. We'd been given all this time – why struggle with existential dread, when you can make banana bread? Everyone announced that they were going to learn Mandarin, do a daily high-intensity interval training (HIIT) workout, or finish their screenplay. I thought of my 'books to read' pile – both the teetering, physical one, quite close now to the light switch and supported, just, by the door frame in my bedroom, and the virtual one of the books I kept promising an imaginary teacher in my head that I'd 'get round to'. Top of the list was the Cazalet Chronicles books, Elizabeth Jane Howard's acclaimed family saga. Their titles did not excite or delight me. The first two books, *The Light Years* and *Marking Time,* sounded as though they were going to be arduous to read.

People I loved and respected kept recommending them forcefully, which made me resent them. It was as though I'd woken up in one of those dreams in which you're made to go back to school, even though you've got a degree and you're in your 30s. Assigned reading had ruined most of my school summer holidays and now it was going to ruin my lockdown too!

I ordered all five of the Cazalet Chronicles, which made me feel earnest, virtuous, and a little weary, the way you might do if you ordered some exercise equipment or a juicer. And, on a drizzly March morning, I picked up book one, *The Light Years,* promising myself that I'd try to read a chapter before I picked up my phone.

When I looked up, the sun was beginning to set and my husband was saying something about dinner. I'd fallen into the book. Living in 2020, at the beginning of the pandemic wasn't much fun. But, strangely, it was fun to visit 1938 and spend time with Louise, Clary, and Polly, who were all holding their breath and waiting for war to break out.

The book had held me. I'd been completely absorbed by the world Howard had created. I'd experienced escapism just when I needed it most. When I was reading, the book felt real. It gave me a break from being Daisy in 2020, confined to her flat and continually refreshing her newsfeed. Instead, I travelled through space and time, ordering cocktails in Edward's club and helping Rachel to get the cousins' bedrooms ready.

However, when I tore myself away from the book, the parallels between the Cazalets' situation and my own weren't lost on me. We were all existing in a suspended state, holding our breath, and waiting. In real life, I noticed that almost every news report used the word 'unprecedented'. There were very few concrete facts and many examples of 'if X, then Y'. Everyone was restless and making guesses. How long would this go on for? How many people would die?

The Cazalets are an imaginary family on the brink of something terrifyingly real. As a reader, I was in the unusual position of knowing the answers to many of their 'ifs' – war *did* break out, it lasted for six years, and no one was untouched by the tragedy, violence, and horror it brought about. It defined a generation. But I was also comforted by the fact that there was a precedent for the 'unprecedented' situation that many of us were in at the start of the pandemic. We were all anxious. We were waiting and we couldn't predict what would happen. We had no idea what the future held. But history – even relatively recent history – was filled with disaster and humans prevailed. And then, just as now, people were still preoccupied by the domestic and the trivial. They had the odd conversation about Chamberlain's strategies and international relations within Europe, but they mostly talked about shopping and meal planning.

In a way, reading about an imaginary family in wartime felt more grounding than consuming the latest news and digital media. It was a much calmer activity. Elizabeth Jane Howard hadn't created a universe that was powered by my clicking and scrolling. Reading was a form of escapism, but it made me feel more measured and informed. It brought context to some complicated circumstances. One of the characters, Villy, frequently says, 'One day we'll all be dead and none of this will matter', echoing the sentiment my mother liked to share when I was a teenager. On first reading, these words frustrated me but, as they were repeated, I started to find them very moving. The next year would be strange and scary, but I'd feel very differently about it in five years' time. And in 500 years, it would be completely forgotten and everyone would be worrying about something else entirely. The only certain thing was that they would be worrying.

Fiction wasn't just more restorative than the news but also seemed to reveal more about the way the world really worked. In the moment, reading allowed me to escape reality at a time when reality felt relentless. It's taught me that no emotion is ever wrong, but some require more management than others.

'Seek help. You deserve it'

To learn more about exactly what anxiety is and how we can manage it, I had a chat with clinical psychologist, neuroscientist, and bestselling author Dr Sophie Mort – AKA Dr Soph. Sophie specialises in taking complex information about our mental health out of medical textbooks and sharing it in a way we can understand and use. She tells me many people look to her to find out more about anxiety and she wants to explain that anxiety itself isn't a problem. But it becomes one when it starts to have an impact on the way we live.

'Anxiety is a natural response to stress or perceived threats, characterised by feelings of worry, nervousness, or unease. It becomes a general issue when it interferes with daily life and persists beyond the challenging situation. Differentiating between logical responses and general issues involves considering how long the symptoms go on for, how intense they are, and how much they are impacting you.'

Sophie says that the way to monitor anxiety is to think about how it is affecting your day-to-day life. 'You may be anxious about something that makes total sense. However, if it is getting in the way of you being able to sleep, eat, concentrate, or do anything you normally do, it has become something that you will benefit from tackling.'

Sophie's understanding of anxiety doesn't just come from her training but also her lived experience. 'I had panic attacks that led me to avoid supermarkets. Avoiding situations that cause anxiety makes sense in the short term. But, in the long term, it means that the next time you try, your symptoms ramp up. Your brain screams "Don't do it, it's too dangerous, you won't cope or survive." In order to get over my supermarket anxiety, I learned breathing exercises as though my life depended on it. Another thing that helped was psychoeducation and learning that anxiety itself is not dangerous. It flows, like a wave, and it will peak and ebb away if you let it.'

Rather than avoiding the situations that make us anxious, Sophie suggests carefully planning our exposure to them, to build up our tolerance and develop coping tools. 'I wrote a step-by-step plan to get back into a supermarket,' she explains. 'The first step was sitting in the car park, breathing until my heart rate settled. The next day I sat near the door for 10 minutes. The next day I stood inside with a friend. We talked and breathed. Just for five minutes. The next day I increased this to 10 minutes. I only increased to the next steps when I knew I could do the one before comfortably.' This advice appeals to me because it's so specific and so practical. We don't have to launch ourselves out of our comfort zones before we're ready, we just keep stretching the edges until the zone is wider and more encompassing.

Sophie explains that when she committed to the plan, it worked. 'Slowly I got to the point I could walk around the supermarket on my own, not sprinting for the door trying to avoid a panic attack. I would feel very anxious, but I would know that it wasn't dangerous and would go if I persisted.' I find this inspiring. It shows that there isn't a 'perfect' solution – anxiety will not be eliminated from our lives – but there are small things we can all do to reduce the impact of anxiety. And by sharing her experiences, Sophie is showing us that anxiety can affect anyone, regardless of how smart and successful they are. Anxiety isn't a sign that we're failing or getting it wrong. In fact, it's a sign that we deserve care. 'It's essential to prioritise self-care, maintain a healthy lifestyle, and reach out for help when needed. When I was 18, and struggling, I got this kind of support. Now I give that support to others. So many people go through this in life and get through this too. Seek help. You deserve it.'

I'm curious about whether Sophie has noticed that reading reduces anxiety – and why she thinks it can be so calming. 'Reading can reduce anxiety by providing a distraction,' she explains, 'but it also fosters a sense of control and mastery.' This makes sense. When I'm absorbed in a story, I feel as though I can understand the world and participate in it at my own pace. Reading reduces my feelings of overwhelm because I'm controlling the flow of information I'm receiving.

Sophie adds, 'Promoting relaxation potentially activates the parasympathetic nervous system.' This is the network of nerves that relaxes your body after periods of stress and danger.[8]   The more we engage the parasympathetic nervous system, the more quickly it calms us and the stronger it becomes.

Sophie also explains that, 'Additionally, engaging in absorbing activities can shift focus away from anxious thoughts and into the present moment.' This makes a lot of sense to me. When I'm overwhelmed by anxiety, it's often because my head is filled with thoughts about the future and I'm worrying about hypothetical situations I have no control over. But when I read – especially in the morning, when I wake up worrying about the day ahead – I find that paying close attention to a book shifts my perspective. I don't avoid my worries but, by changing where I'm placing my attention and my energy, I have a stronger understanding of what I can and can't control. Like Sophie in the supermarket, I know that some anxiety might still be present, but I can cope with it.

Five ways to get yourself to pick up a book when you're feeling anxious

• **Try returning to the beginning of your reading journey**
On the You're Booked podcast, I always ask guests if they
can remember the first book they chose to read and loved – the
story that wasn't given to them by a parent or a teacher but felt
as though it was truly *theirs*. Can you remember yours? It doesn't
need to be complicated or sophisticated – maybe it was one of
the Twilight, Magic Faraway Tree series or Elmer books. Have a
look for a copy (it doesn't have to be expensive – you could
request and reserve it from your local library or AbeBooks is a
great online source of second-hand titles). Make a little ritual out
of reading it, as though you were meditating. You only need 10
minutes, but try to find somewhere calm and quiet, where you
won't be disturbed. Hopefully, when you start reading, you'll feel
as though you're being reunited with some old friends. You'll
also be reunited with some emotions. The familiar story will

bring back a sense of connection, focus, comfort, and joy. A lot of anxiety stems from a fear of uncertainty and the unknown. Returning to a book you know well will ease your anxiety and make the reading experience feel secure.

• **You don't need to be a physical book purist** There are so many ways to read, and so many reasons why a traditional print book might not be the best fit for you. Angela, a friend with mobility issues, tells me, 'Most hardbacks are too heavy for me to hold for very long, but I can read much more comfortably with a Kindle.' The only rule is that you read in a way that suits you. If you're a big podcast listener, audiobooks are perfect for you. I read in all formats. Sometimes, if I'm struggling to put my phone down, I pick up my e-reader, which gives me the sensation of being on a device, but gives me a single thing to focus on instead of infinite things.

• **Be patient and be as kind to yourself as you can** But try to be kind to reading too. Remember, you've spent your adult life training your brain to sprint. Now you're asking it to try cross-country running. You have all the right skills, but it might take a few goes to remember how to use them.

• **Start with your special interests** Think about the themes and subjects that really light you up and look for the books that match them. If you're a true crime podcast fiend, look for crime novels and psychological thrillers. If you adored *Bridgerton* on Netflix, I've got great news – there's a whole series of books waiting for you. Whether you're a cook, gardener, football obsessive, make-up junkie, there's a book about your specialist subject. (I have been known to take recipe books to bed and read them as though they're novels – especially anything by Nigella Lawson or Diana Henry.)

• **When building any habit, the way to do it is little and often** You don't have to read every single day, but the more you do it – even 10 minutes at a time – the more you'll *want* to do it and the sooner you'll feel the incredible benefits. Reading regularly has been proved to make your brain stronger (some studies have shown that reading and other mental exercises can slow or prevent dementia), as well as reduce stress by up to 68 per cent (according to a study in 2009 at the University of Sussex).[9] It's like any other exercise – there are days when it makes us feel better, almost instantly, and days when it feels impossible in the moment, but we feel wonderful afterwards. Over time, the rewards will start to stack up.

Brilliant books for managing anxiety

A Manual for Being Human by Dr Sophie Mort

A wise, compassionate guide that will help you to make sense of some of your most complex, painful emotions, and to treat yourself with kindness.

Almost Everything by Anne Lamott

A generous and gentle essay collection that explores some of the trickiest and most overwhelming aspects of being a human. It's worth getting a copy for these words alone: 'Almost everything will work again if you unplug it for a few minutes, including you.'[10]

'Life doesn't frighten me' by Maya Angelou

This electric, inspiring poem is for everyone who is or has ever been a child. It's about accepting the presence of fear and recognising the weight of our own power. The version of it published as a book for children and illustrated with Jean Michel-Basquiat's paintings is beautiful.

2

Read yourself SECURE

"All the reading she had done had given her a view of life they had never seen"

Roald Dahl[1]

The Spice Girls are on the radio and half the class is singing along. A paper aeroplane flies past my head. I can hear screams of laughter. Everyone else is in a brilliant mood. No one has noticed me, sitting by myself. No one is coming to comfort me. Even though I'm in a room full of people, I feel lonely. I don't fit in here. I know what I ought to do. Perhaps I'd have some friends if I could pull myself together and make an effort to smile and speak to people. But I feel too insecure to try. I don't have anything to offer anyone. I'm not good at anything.

I'm holding my half-term school report and holding back my tears. The one thing I'm not holding back is self-pity. It's streaming from my pores. You could knit a jumper out of it. I'm convinced that I'll never be happy again. Everything is going wrong. Half-term starts tomorrow, so I should be in a great mood, but all I can think about is this report. 'Daisy tries hard.' 'Daisy does her best.' But Daisy doesn't do as well as her classmates. Daisy gets Bs. And the odd C. Daisy doesn't have anything going for her. She isn't sporty. She isn't popular. She isn't thin. She wears the wrong clothes – she's the only girl who turned up on non-uniform day in her school shoes.

At my old school, I didn't mind the fact that I wasn't sporty or popular. I was happy to be quiet and nerdy. I got As, but I didn't think it was a big deal – it was my thing. Everyone had a thing! I would have gladly swapped with Laura Kerins, whose thing was being stepcousins with Joe from *EastEnders*, but at least I had an identity. I felt secure there. As a nerd, I had a job, a role, something holding me in place.

I'd been so excited about starting my new school – a girls' grammar. Rumour had it that everyone here was quiet and nerdy – weird in the specific way that I was weird. I thought I'd feel normal at last!

However, it turns out that, at grammar school, everyone else somehow gets straight As without being a massive nerd. They are also pretty, sporty, and much thinner than me. Here, I'm a nobody. I don't matter. I'm mediocre. I'm just *drifting*. No one can see me. Now I have printed proof of this, and I must go home and show it to my parents. Aged 12, I can say with absolute certainty that I will never amount to anything.

Comparison crisis

I suspect we all fantasise about going back in time and having a chat with our Past Selves. We'd all love to tell our young ghosts that heartbreak doesn't last for ever, no one on their deathbed ever wishes they'd skipped more desserts, and we probably don't need to own more than one sequinned blazer at a time. I'd like to give that 12-year-old the biggest hug – but I'd also like to tell her to lighten up.

She was waiting for someone or something to make her feel secure. I wish she'd known that it wouldn't come from outside; she had to work on feeling it from within. 'Young Daisy, I guarantee you that every other girl in this room has felt this way or will feel this way in the future. I promise that no one who feels happy or secure in themselves would ever make fun of someone else's shoes. You're somebody! And you're *12 years old*. You're still discovering what makes you you. But you won't find it by comparing yourself with everyone else, and you certainly won't find it in your school report.'

At the time, I made it into a Scarlet O'Hara moment. With God as my witness, I would never be found imperfect again! During the half-term holiday, I started to hatch a plan. With diet, exercise, and *really* hard work, I'd be safe. I didn't think I could ever be the best – I just wanted to stop feeling like the worst. I reasoned that if I made myself more acceptable, other people would accept me and I'd never feel insecure again.

It never occurred to me that I might be a perfectionist; I wasn't perfect enough to be one. But I internalised the idea that being less than perfect was unforgivable. My peers did too.

I should point out that we were privileged. Our teachers were universally kind, patient, and encouraging. They wanted us to fulfil our potential and they believed that potential was considerable. If we were struggling, they'd help us. No one got locked in a cupboard for getting a C. No one was encouraging us to compete and compare ourselves with one another. And yet we all did it, all the time.

The stress of school drove me to develop some unhealthy coping mechanisms. I abused food – starving myself, bingeing, and purging – believing that if I had a smaller body, everything else would fall into place. When I was 15, I fainted at the bottom of a hill during a run. I was almost run over by a car. Luckily, the driver saw me and stopped in time. I was taken to hospital. Even then, it didn't occur to me that I was hurting myself and being thinner wasn't going to change anything. I believed that making my body smaller would make me feel more secure; instead, it made me feel even more invisible.

Schoolwork became another obsession. At my old school I'd been 'the clever one', so I thought if I could claim my old identity in this new school, maybe it'd be the way I could fit in. I just had to work much harder. I started my homework as soon as it was set and I was obsessive about achieving, and maintaining, top marks. I didn't ever feel proud of myself; I felt scared about what might happen if I slipped or stopped. I ate and slept very little. I was exhausted.

But I had books. Reading gave me a glimmer of a life beyond my obsessive routine. When I read, I could relax. Stories gave me a sense of yearning, glamour, and adventure. They stoked my imagination and made me believe that, while the present was hard, there might be hope and fun in my future. Most importantly, when I read a book, I felt seen and understood. Reading brought me the sense of security I craved. I didn't have to jostle with anyone else or justify my place in the world when I was lost in a book. As a reader, I felt as though I'd been invited to wander around in someone else's imagination for as long as I liked.

In my English classes, I fell in love with poetry. That was the only place where I genuinely didn't care about my marks. Reading T. S. Eliot and Tennyson transported me to a brighter, more vivid world where exams didn't matter. And in real life, I wasn't as pretty or popular as Amy, Kirsty, or Emma, but I could find plenty of imaginary friends – Cassandra Mortmain from *I Capture the Castle,* the Robinson family from the Gemma series, Olivia Curtis from *Invitation to the Waltz.* At school, I was certain that I was the saddest, loneliest, weirdest girl in the building. But at home, alone in bed, I'd open the book under my pillow and those feelings of loneliness would dissolve. According to my books, there *were* other people out there who felt just like me. They didn't go to my school, but I might meet them one day.

Social comparison theory

The ironic thing about loneliness is that we're all in it together. It affects everyone at times, and it's on the rise. In 2022, the Campaign to End Loneliness reported that, in the UK, almost half of us have some feelings of loneliness, with 7.1 per cent – 3.83 million people – in Great Britain reporting 'chronic loneliness', experiencing feelings of loneliness 'often or always' (up from 6 per cent in 2020).[2]

Nearly everyone will experience loneliness at some point. In 2021, the results of a survey of British adults by an international team of psychologists were published and they found that 'upward social comparisons predicted current loneliness'.[3] Personally, I've found that the two are intertwined. I don't necessarily feel lonely when I am alone, but the moment I start comparing myself with my peers, I feel isolated, as well as inadequate. I can spend a happy afternoon reading alone and I'll feel connected and content. But if I put my book down and scroll through Instagram, I find that I start telling myself stories. I can see two friends together and wonder whether I've been deliberately excluded from something fun. I can see someone else's achievement and immediately make their result mean something about my lack of attainment. When I read a book on a bad day, I feel better and I'm quickly completely immersed in a world that has nothing to do with me. When I look at social media on a bad day, I start to construct horror stories and I'm starring in every one of them.

We've never had more ways to communicate with one another and be in touch, but is social media making us lonely? And how can reading help?

In 1954, social psychologist Leon Festinger proposed the concept of social comparison theory (SCT).[4] He suggested that we all tend to look to our peers so we can glean an understanding of our own status – especially when it comes to our strengths and abilities. Festinger's research showed that these kinds of comparisons are part of being human. It's possible that we all started to become more aware of this tendency to compare in the 50s, following the Second World War. As the Western world returned to peace and prosperity, a growing number of people were starting to experience greater freedom of choice in work and leisure, and they had more disposable income to spend. Class barriers started to shift. Perhaps it seemed a little easier to look over the fence and wonder whether the neighbour's lawn was greener than ours.

Some 50 years after Festinger introduced his theory, the very first version of Facebook was launched, and our curtain twitching was digitised. At the time of writing, we have access to a huge amount of information about our 'neighbours' – global as well as local. We can know everything that anyone chooses to share about their work, wardrobe, holidays, family, finances, and food choices. But access to all this information has various effects on us. The Royal Society for Public Health and Young Health Movement reported in 2017 that using Snapchat, Facebook, Instagram and Twitter (now X) increased feelings of depression, anxiety, poor body image, and loneliness among adolescents in the UK.[5] Other studies have found that social media use can result in disrupted sleep,[6] which reduces the quality of our physical and mental health, and it can exacerbate social anxiety.[7]

We all know this. Many of us are trying to cut down on our social media use and screen time. My friend Sara, 48, tells me that being the parent of a teenager has made her increasingly aware of her own digital habits. 'My daughter is 15, and we've both noticed that being online can exacerbate her anxiety. We're also both starting to realise that she's grown up watching me continually using my phone, and she's seen how often I reach for it and how much it affects me. I would say she's probably got a much healthier relationship with social media than I have – she's quick to notice how it makes her feel and she puts it down.'

Sara adds, 'Perhaps ironically, one of my biggest social media struggles is that I compare my parenting with other parents!' When I see that other mums have organised amazing holidays and trips, and their children are always engaged in wholesome, outdoorsy activities, I feel as though I'm not good enough as a mother. It's my daughter who is quick to remind me that we're not seeing the whole picture. She tells me that if she's having a great time, she forgets to take pictures. She's the one who says, "It's ironic that it's called social media because it makes me feel really lonely!"'

Perhaps we should all pay attention to Sara's daughter's words. For me, loneliness and comparison seem to go hand in hand. When I look at what everyone else is doing, I feel left out and inadequate. When I use social media, there's a bottomless well of 'everyone else'. In the space of five minutes, I can compare myself with an old friend from primary school, my neighbour, my cousin, Alexandria Ocasio-Cortez, and Taylor Swift. And no matter how many times I tell myself that nothing good can come of it and these people are probably also comparing themselves with one another, it's very hard to stop.

My mother, who is in her 60s, has an interesting perspective on this. 'I don't want to bore on about "the good old days", but I think a little boringness might be what's missing for all of us. On a typical Sunday in the 70s, there was *nothing to do*. My family would go to church, we'd have lunch, and then that was it. Barely anything on TV, even. I read books then because that was my favourite form of entertainment. But I think it helped that I knew absolutely everyone else was in the same boat. Without having a place to look and check, all my friends were at home, reading or being bored, and probably helping with the washing-up. I don't know how I would have concentrated on a book if I'd had Instagram and just known that there was a place I could go and check what everyone else was up to.'

Without realising, my mother was cultivating a habit that has been proven to fight feelings of loneliness. In the short term, picking up a book and losing yourself in a story is going to be much more fun than picking up your phone and wishing you had someone else's thighs or bank account. But in the long term, reading and reducing those feelings of loneliness could have a huge impact on your physical and mental health. Several studies, including one published by the Queen's Reading Room in 2024, have found that high-frequency readers are less likely to experience different kinds of loneliness, and reducing loneliness reduces the likelihood of dementia.[8]

As a teenager, I was relentlessly critical of myself, determined to achieve and excel, and to win everyone's approval. I was also *completely* self-obsessed. (This is a common part of adolescent development. A study in 2006 found that teenagers use the superior temporal sulcus part of the brain – not the prefrontal cortex – to make decisions,[9] which means that they are less able to understand how their actions might affect others than adults.) Back then, my loneliness could trigger feelings of extreme self-pity – everything was 'the worst' and everything was about me. How I loved hyperbole! But if I was reading, I couldn't feel sorry for myself for long. Fiction made other people's tragedies and challenges very real to me.

Reading can help us to develop empathy. In 2015, the findings of a study by psychologist Diana Tamir and her fellow researchers revealed that reading fiction often improves people's 'social cognition' and strengthens their ability to empathise with and understand what the people around them are thinking and feeling.[10] This makes sense to me as the more I read, the more I learn that we all have secret struggles, moments of shame and embarrassment, and dreams we daren't mention out loud.

Diaries of... somebodies

If I'm feeling lonely, longing for intimacy, and craving an antidote to the feelings of despair I sometimes get after a prolonged Instagram session, I like to read someone else's diary. I don't mean that I let myself into someone's home and go through their bedside drawers. Instead, I find an old friend on my bookshelf – *Bridget Jones's Diary*, *The Secret Diary of Adrian Mole Aged 13¾*, or *The Diary of a Nobody*. Diary novels are the perfect cure for when you've been comparing yourself with everyone else because they make it clear you're not the only person in the world with an internal monologue that seems to be out of control.

Adrian Mole is a fictional character, but he's loved by so many readers because his thoughts and feelings seem so real to us. We read the books, we see ourselves, and we laugh at ourselves. We've all felt insecure. We've all experienced romantic rejection. We've all worried that no one takes us seriously. We've all fought with our parents and we have all worried about money. When I read the words of this character, I feel as though I can laugh at myself and with myself. I also feel empathy for my fellow readers. This makes me feel secure. I know I'm in good company because thousands of other people have read and loved these books and found themselves in them like me. When we laugh at Adrian, we're laughing at ourselves too. Meeting a fellow Adrian Mole fan is liberating because it usually means that here is someone who has the same secret anxieties as me and a similar sense of humour.

It can be hard to talk frankly about our greatest vulnerabilities and seek reassurance from our friends, but there are books that make it easier. When I first read *Bridget Jones's Diary,* I was 13. I understood that it was a satire and it was skewering particular aspects of the British middle classes with wicked specificity. I realised that it was a smart retelling of *Pride and Prejudice* and drawing smart parallels between attitudes towards love and marriage in the 18th century and the 20th century. I could see that if the story had a 'moral', it was that we should all stop exhausting ourselves with endless quests for self-improvement and just be.

However, I also felt as though the universe had created a brand-new best friend expressly for me and delivered her to the local library. Bridget had a gang, and I felt as included by her friends (Jude, Shazzer, Tom, and Magda) as I felt excluded by the girls at school. When I read the words, 'Being a woman is worse than being a farmer. There is so much harvesting and crop spraying to be done: legs to be waxed, underarms shaved, eyebrows plucked, feet pumiced, skin exfoliated and moisturised, spots cleansed, roots dyed, eyelashes tinted, nails filed, cellulite massaged, stomach muscles exercised,'[11] I laughed out loud and felt my shoulders dropping. I found it so funny because I was starting to realise that I was expected to perform an ever-growing litany of 'lady chores' and I was wondering whether there was something really, really wrong with me. Surely no one was supposed to be quite as lumpy, hairy, and unpolished-looking as I was? Bridget was the first person to tell me that looking 'natural' actually required a lot of thankless work. Tiring, time-consuming, expensive work that never, ever feels as though it's completed. As I read, an idea lodged itself in my mind. I started to suspect that, secretly, everyone felt imperfect and that being perfect isn't very interesting, anyway.

Some years later, when I was in my 20s, the universe delivered another brand-new best friend to me, this time in real life – or something like it. I 'met' Lauren online when her brother Dan tagged me and tweeted, 'Lauren, this girl sounds exactly like you.' We met for a drink and discovered, quite quickly, that our respective adolescences and all our expectations of adult life had been shaped by Bridget Jones. Our experiences were spookily similar. We read our books in semi-secret, looking out for them in local libraries and charity shops, knowing our parents probably wouldn't approve.

We didn't love the book for its love story, but for the way it made the world sharp and soft. It mocked the offices we hoped to work in and the dinner parties we hoped we might be invited to – it made our understanding of adulthood more vivid and less frightening.

Its critics have accused the book, the character, and the author, Helen Fielding, of promoting poor body image and spreading an unfeminist message – that marriage is the ultimate goal for women. But it had the opposite effect on both Lauren and me. As teenagers, we looked forward to finding our own 'urban family' and developing strong adult friendships. We didn't dream of finding Mr Darcy (although I'll confess to a crush on Mr Wrong, Daniel Cleaver), we read it as a cautionary tale about marriage. Bridget's mother briefly leaves Bridget's father and he's devastated. Bridget's 'smug married' friends have mostly made appalling matches – Bridget doesn't want to trade places with anyone at the dinner parties. Magda, the friend who has it all, discovers that her husband, Jeremy, is having an affair.

I think the book is a hymn to imperfection on every level. Being 'thin' won't save us. Marriage won't save us. The dream job won't save us. I often think of *Bridget Jones's Diary* when I see influencers and celebrities announcing their divorces not long after posting a series of glossy photos and videos sharing moments from their 'perfect' family life. When we feel insecure about being imperfect, it's easy to briefly construct and post an outer layer of perfection. Sometimes we can find more truths about ourselves in fiction than we're able to share on social media or out loud.

Lauren introduced me to Bridget Jones's spiritual predecessor – E. M. Delafield's *Diary of a Provincial Lady*, and I found another friend. This book is also about being an imperfect person, trying one's best, and attempting to get on top of everything, but petty grievances and annoyances get in the way. It's the diary of a woman in her mid-30s, living in Devon, with two children and a vaguely exasperating husband. There's enough money for a cook and a housekeeper, but not sufficient to stop her always feel vaguely self-conscious about the shabbiness of her dresses, and she finds herself travelling to the next town to pawn her best jewellery. It's self-effacing, but never self-pitying, and it taught me that some of the best protection against comparison and perfectionism involves developing a sense of humour about yourself. After all, who would want to be the joyless, bossy, Lady Boxe? (If you've not read it, she always knows exactly how things should be done, but waits to share that information until they have been done the wrong way!)

Slowly, via my bookshelves, I began to realise that the quest to be the best doesn't leave us much room for growth. When we compare ourselves with other people, we stop being curious about them. We assume they know better, and that they are better. We don't stop to ask what their challenges are or look to see how we can help. When I compare myself with other people, it exacerbates my tendency to make everything about *me*. But when I read about fictional lives, it makes me more curious about people's real lives because I've gained an insight into human interiority. I believe that curiosity can make us all kinder, wiser, and stronger.

'We're not binary... Relish those shades of grey'

Someone who knows a lot about confidence, comparison, and perfectionism – and how the latter can have impacts on the former – is bestselling author, coach, podcaster, and Amazing If co-founder, Sarah Ellis. Sarah and her business partner, Helen Tupper, specialise in helping people with their 'squiggly careers', and have given a very successful TEDTalk, 'The best career path isn't always a straight line'.[12] Sarah explains that she can see how comparison culture and perfectionism have an enormous emotional impact on all of us and can stop us from exploring our unique potential.

Sarah says, 'We can't underestimate how stressful our lives are now. We are *constantly* being presented with information about everyone we've ever met. The first thing to mention is that we need to forgive ourselves for our perfectionism instead of fighting it – especially when it comes to the way we use social media and read the news. The information is formatted, purposively, to be addictive. We can't necessarily cut ourselves off from it, and we don't have to. But we can cultivate spaces that are separate from it. I love reading because it gives me some respite from a very noisy online life. The nature of my work means that I can't be a digital hermit, I've got to throw myself into the noise. But I can protect my reading time. It's a hobby that engages my brain and gives me a chance to escape.'

When I spoke with Sarah, she and Helen were working on a project called 'Caging your confidence gremlins'. It's about giving us the keys we need to understand what has an impact on our confidence in particular and how we can make sure our individual gremlins stay locked in the cage, not get out and wreak havoc in our life. I tell Sarah that comparison is my biggest, most frightening gremlin. 'You can look at it in terms of zoom-in, zoom-out thinking,' Sarah explains. 'Sometimes it's useful to look at a problem in detail and really focus, but zooming out and seeing a fuller picture will give you a wider context and make the experience of comparison less intense. Firstly, we all know this, but it's absolutely fine to make life easier for yourself. Everyone has a right to share their lives online. Equally, you have the right to mute and unfollow. You don't have to tell anyone that you're doing it. Keeping up with everyone's news on Facebook and Instagram can feel like a second job. If it's bringing up complicated feelings, it's fine to opt out of that.'

I realise that, for me, the medium can affect the message. If a close friend shares their exciting news in person, it feels like part of an intimate conversation, and any envy or jealousy I feel is usually overshadowed by happiness for them. If I learn of their exciting news on social media, I immediately compare their achievements with mine, and find myself lacking. I believe I'm an empathetic person, so why do I find it so hard to locate that empathy when I'm online? And could boosting my empathy stop me from comparing myself with everyone else?

Sarah says, 'Firstly, we're not binary. We're allowed to be complex and inconsistent. It's completely natural and human to compare, and to feel jealous, envious, and inadequate. The feelings aren't wrong. They're only a problem when they start to overshadow your happiness and stop you from doing the things you want to do. You could easily compare yourself with plenty of other people and discover that they all have very similar emotional responses when it comes to comparison. This isn't black and white. Relish those shades of grey. This is a very nuanced area, which brings us back to fiction. I love fiction because it's filled with nuance. In the business book world, nuance doesn't necessarily sell. Everyone loves the idea of things like "Five Steps to Becoming a CEO". We're all looking for the quickest, straightest path possible but, more often than not, that's not the right path for us.'

Sarah's words make me realise why I have a tendency to compare, and despair, when I look at social media. It's a great place to showcase big achievements, but we can't always see how those milestones were achieved. We assume everyone has taken a very straight path to success because we can't see the nuance.

'When I read fiction, I'm reminded of how important it is to really spend time in other people's worlds,' says Sarah. 'Reading stories has been proven, time and time again, to boost our empathy. We get a much fuller picture of human experience in a novel than we do on social media. I think there's an emotional realness to it, even though the events described didn't actually happen. Fiction can help us to bridge the gap and understand the depth of another person's experience, beyond what they're able to tell us or show us.'

However, Sarah is the first to explain that, while her book habit has considerable benefits for her business, she reads for pleasure first – and she thinks it's important to be selfish. 'I believe that making time to read just for fun, and just for me, makes me happier, stronger, and much more resilient. It doesn't matter what your gremlins are, doing something that's just for you will make it easier to cage them.'

She adds, 'It sounds as though reading directly helps your perfectionist tendencies and your problems with comparison by making you more empathetic, but I think the fact that you can lose yourself in a book and find joy in stories will help you to recover more quickly from a bout of comparison. There's an author called Alex Soojung-Kim Pang who talks about the importance of active rest. This could be cooking, or gardening – reading is my favourite form of active rest. The idea is that you're fully immersed in something, but you're present. You're taking part in an activity that requires some engagement from you.

Finding a little time in your day for some form of active rest will boost your resilience and help you to handle the gremlins, wobbles, and problems you come up against. This has been the best side effect of my reading habit. We all get distracted; it's hard for us all to pay attention. A book doesn't give us the same instant gratification that a phone does, but we can find pleasure in a book – it just takes a bit of practice.'

Ultimately, what does Sarah suggest that we do? 'Firstly, cut yourself some slack. The first step to understanding our perfectionism is to remind ourselves that we don't have to be emotionally perfect. It's normal to compare ourselves with our peers, and it's normal to feel bad about it. Sometimes, simply accepting our emotional state is the first step to feeling better.'

She adds, 'Next, see if there's anything you can do to make life a bit easier. If you'd be happier muting or unfollowing some accounts, then by all means do so. But I think the way to make a long-term change is by thinking about active rest. It doesn't have to be a reading habit but, for me, reading has brought so many unexpected long-term benefits. I'm calmer, happier, and better at paying attention. This means that I can spot and tame my confidence gremlins as they're escaping and stop them before they start to cause havoc. And if you are struggling with comparison, reading and strengthening your sense of empathy will really help.'

Cures for comparison anxiety

So, how can we stop comparison from holding us back? And where does reading come in?

• **Frustratingly, the first step lies in accepting that it can't be 'cured'** There's no book, no expert, and no combination of tips to follow that will stop you from comparing yourself with anyone else ever again – it's a natural human response. When it bubbles up, try to remember that, even though it feels so isolating, people all over the world are experiencing the same emotions as you. You feel 'wrong' but that doesn't mean something is wrong with you.

• **Reading can help in the long term** Think of it as fixing your roof when the sun is shining. When you're feeling relaxed, confident, and energetic, investing that energy in boosting your mental health will really help when it starts raining. Reading from a book every day – ideally fiction – has been shown to boost your empathy, increase your attention span, and reduce feelings of loneliness. You're fuelling your happiness tank, so when painful feelings arise, you'll feel stronger and better equipped to deal with them.

• **Reading can help in the short term too** The more you read, the more you'll recognise what you crave from stories and the better you'll get at selecting the books that will bring you the comfort and release you need. You might need a sobering book to put your feelings in perspective, for example. I recently got over some comparison woes pretty quickly when I picked up *In Memoriam* by Alice Winn, which is about the plight of young, closeted men dying in the First World War. But when I was feeling blue about work and comparing myself with other writers, *Yellowface* by Rebecca F. Kuang, was the wickedly satirical antidote to my self-pity. It's a great cautionary tale about the perils of comparing yourself with your most successful friends.

• **Think about what builds your feelings of empathy and what reduces those feelings** I notice that when I spend a lot of time on social media, I feel alienated from my friends and burned out by an information overload. It robs me of a feeling of shared intimacy and experiencing goals and milestones with them. But the more I read, the more I build my sense of what other people's lives are really like and I don't have to rely on seeing what they post. Also, nothing boosts a friendship or bonds me to someone like comparing notes on a book we've both loved. It makes me feel connected, not isolated – and the more connected I feel, the less likely I am to find myself comparing and despairing.

Books to shore us up

The Trebizon Boarding School series by Anne Digby

Any series of school stories will do the trick for me, but I have a very soft spot for these novels about a fictional school in Cornwall, with young girls growing up and finding their place in the world. Whenever I read the Trebizon books, I feel as though I'm part of a special gang.

Wow, No Thank You by Samantha Irby

I love this extremely funny essay collection because Irby celebrates and cheers for all the parts of myself I try to push away – my tiredness, grumpiness, tendency towards IBS. She makes perfectionism seem pointless, and her humour and warmth create real intimacy. When I read these books, I feel connected.

Wintering by Katherine May

This is the perfect book to reach for whenever you're feeling quiet and sad. It's about the fact that rest is *vital*, and it's a guide to finding ways to nurture and nourish yourself when you're feeling estranged from yourself. When I pick this up, I remember that my disconnected, lonely feeling is usually just exhaustion and, when I read Katherine's words, I can start to build the space I need to rest.

3
Read yourself
FUNNIER

"Have a depressed feeling that this is going to be another case of *Orlando* about which was perfectly able to talk most intelligently until I read it and found myself unfortunately unable to understand any of it"

E. M. Delafield[1]

I am hysterical. Giddy, gleeful, and completely powerless over the waves of laughter that keep breaking out of me. The sheer silliness of the situation keeps presenting itself to me anew. I've given myself to the spirit of this book; I'm high. There's something elegant about the way logic and reason have become unravelled. I don't ever want to stop laughing.

The book is called *The Incredible Adventures of Professor Branestawm*. It was a Christmas present, but it's been sitting on the shelf unread until I reached for it in a moment of boredom during the school holidays.

Professor Branestawm is an inventor, a 'mad scientist', and an absent-minded genius. His brilliant inventions and high-concept plans mean that he struggles to function and complete everyday tasks. In my young brain, I can relate. And I think that Branestawm's invention of an inflatable pocket motor car is one of the cleverest ideas I've ever come across. It doesn't require petrol, which seems ideal. The hole in the ozone layer keeps being mentioned on the kids' current affairs show, *Newsround*, and sometimes I worry about it so much that I can't get to sleep. I'm also anxious every time we go on a family car journey because of the inordinate amount of stress and rage that is unleashed whenever my father is tasked with finding a parking space. There always seems to be a genuine risk of never being able to leave the car and having to circle the car park for the rest of our lives.

But there's a very good reason why the Professor's invention isn't a long-term solution to these issues. And when I find out what it is, I'm laughing too hard to worry. The explosion in the drawing pin factory is delicious. I can hear the pins raining down. I can picture the bewildered motorists, sitting on the road in shock as their cars collapse around them. And I can laugh at the idea of the whole Pagwell area (Great Pagwell, Little Pagwell, Pagwell Heights, Pagwell Gardens, Lower Pagwell, Upper Pagwell, Pagwell Green, Pagwell Centre, Pagwell Marke, and Pagwell Dock) being brought to a halt by a shower of pins. There's something very funny about a giant factory being used to make something so small and insignificant.

The drawing pins are powerful. They have brought me so much joy. This book has turned a light on inside my head. I feel in thrall to something wonderful, something bigger and better than anything that scares me. I've read funny books before and I laugh at things I see on TV. I hear jokes at school. But I usually feel, at best, amused. A lot of 'funny' things go over my head. I realise that I love this book because it's absurd. It takes its silliness very seriously. There's a consistency to the Professor Branestawm universe – it runs on its own solid logic and I adore it. Its funniness is an ocean that I want to stay submerged in.

Are you not entertained?

I realise there's no bad feeling that laughter can't cure, at least briefly. When I need a hit of silly weirdness, I return to Professor Branestawm again. It's the gateway drug that eventually leads me to P. G. Wodehouse, Sue Townsend, Sophie Kinsella, Helen Fielding, E. M. Delafield, David Nicholls, Marian Keyes, David Sedaris, Nora Ephron, and Samantha Irby. In time, it will have an enormous influence on my own writing. I'll learn that laughter is one of the best parts of being alive. I seek out the absurd and celebrate it. I stop worrying about the fact that I find the 'wrong' things funny, and some jokes will raise a smile, but other things

– exploding, inflatable cars, Sideshow Bob stepping on a seemingly endless succession of rakes, the sight of Julie Walters in a tabard, Rik Mayall and Ade Edmondson whacking each other's faces with frying pans – will make me weep, honk, and hiccup. I will never, ever apologise for my stupid sense of humour – because it lights up my life. And when a different ocean is threatening to take me and the waves are crashing over my head, I'll look to anything that might make me laugh to stop despair from setting in.

In that search, we don't always look to books. Reading is supposed to be a serious business. Are we being educated if we're also being entertained? When we consider literature, we're disinclined to take comedy seriously. And it's wholly subjective. One person's 'laugh-out-loud must-read' might leave you cold. Parts of *Middlemarch* made me giggle, but I've never been able to enjoy the jokes in a Terry Pratchett book. (Pratchett fans, I know you're legion and I can *hear* you shaking your heads and saying, 'But you laughed at *drawing pins*.' I know. I don't get it, either.)

According to the awards and prize committees, not all funny books are equal. I'm always over the moon when a funny book breaks through. When *Less* by Andrew Sean Greer won the Pulitzer Prize for Fiction in 2018, comedy fans were delighted – and amazed. In the *Washington Post*, book critic Ron Charles wrote, 'What makes this year's winner so unusual is that his novel is funny. *Very funny*. Laugh-till-you-can't-breathe funny. That just doesn't happen in the hallowed chambers of literary honor. Pulitzers are endowed on funereal novels like Cormac McCarthy's *The Road* or cerebral books like Marilynne Robinson's *Gilead*.'[2] To the readers who love to laugh, Greer's achievement felt like a benediction. Comedy was being taken seriously. This was a book that wasn't dark, daunting, or obfuscating – it welcomed its readers and, for once, our taste was deemed literary and worthy.

Greer himself said he had intended to write a serious novel about being gay and ageing, 'But after a year, I just couldn't do it. It sounds strange, but what I was writing about was so sad to me that I thought the only way to write about this is to make it a funny story. And I found that by making fun of myself, I could actually get closer to real emotion – closer to what I wanted in my more serious books.'[3] *Less* is a complex and compelling love story, and Greer uses humour to show the depth of his hero, Arthur Less. He finds himself in increasingly absurd situations. He becomes vulnerable and frustrated. We laugh with him and we feel for him.

Another triumph for comic writing came in 2022, when Percival Everett's shocking novel *The Trees* was shortlisted for the Booker Prize. It's a satire of pulp fiction, a revenge fantasy – a gruesome, gripping exploration of crime and racism in Mississippi. *The Trees* is as disturbing as it is funny, and Everett uses humour to subvert our expectations and draw our attention to racism, bigotry, and intergenerational trauma. I loved the book and laughed loud and often. The twisted comedy makes the book propulsive and compulsive, pulling the reader into and through the story. But reading it made me feel anxious and uncomfortable. Should I be laughing at this? Was I allowed to? This is the power of satire. Everett's bold, vital book reminded me of exactly why we need to take comedy seriously. It's a strong force. If *The Trees* hadn't made me laugh, I might have struggled to pick it up and absorb its message. If it hadn't shown racism at its most laughably grotesque, it wouldn't have stayed with me in the same way. Its comedy comes with a call to action: once I'd laughed at the book, I couldn't ignore its message.

But there's still a lot of snobbery that surrounds funny fiction and I think it's coming between some excellent books and us, the readers, who need them the most. Being lost in a book that makes you laugh is a delicious balm for an anxious day. But when critics dismiss or ignore some of the funniest books, it's harder for us to find them. The Bollinger Everyman Wodehouse Prize for comic fiction has been accused of sexism, with just three women winning it in 18 years.

I'm hugely grateful to writer, actor, and comic Helen Lederer, who set up the Comedy Women In Print Prize (CWIP). Lederer's prize celebrates all forms of funny fiction and dares to challenge a lot of the prejudice and pretension that surrounds the label 'literary'. In her memoir, *Not That I'm Bitter*, Lederer wrote that the act of creating the prize, and a space to celebrate women and comedy, eased some of her fear and tension: 'Witty women's writing is finally on the map, and for now, at least, there's an absence of anxiety.'[4]

The books I turn to over and over again are the ones that reliably make me laugh. And if I'm torn between two books, I'll always pick the one that looks funniest. For me, there's something generous and inclusive about a funny book. Perhaps this is because so much humour is drawn from our humanity and vulnerability. We laugh with characters when they remind us of ourselves and make us feel a little less frail and foolish. And while humour can be used to shock, subvert, and twist our expectations, sometimes funny books can simply make us feel better. Laughing boosts our mental and physical health – when we laugh, we take in more oxygen and we improve our circulation. We release endorphins, and some research suggests that laughing improves our ability to withstand pain.[5]

Old friends

According to research, we're 30 times more likely to laugh out loud in a group than when we're alone.[6] Also, when we read, we need to work harder to get to the gag. Finding humour in a book is an active experience. We have to find and understand double meanings, create our own audiovisual experience and bring the joke to life. It seems improbable that any of us would ever laugh out loud by ourselves, with a book, but I do it all the time.

I often laugh to myself remembering a scene in Kingsley Amis's *Lucky Jim,* when Dixon has lied about his ability to sight-read music and finds himself forced to sing madrigals. We've all been in situations where a white lie or a mistake has got out of hand and we've been vulnerable to it being exposed. And the stakes are high – Dixon needs to impress his colleagues – but we're laughing at his hubris, while also relating to his brittle vulnerability. When I read that book, and laugh for the hundredth time, I feel as though I'm reminiscing with an old friend. That's why I often read my favourite funny books in the early hours of the morning, when I can't sleep. I never have to face my 4am fears alone when I can pick up a book and find a friend with a funny story.

'If a book doesn't make me laugh, I don't feel bad about dropping it'

I wanted to know what makes a funny book and how we find the books that will make us laugh, so I interviewed my friend Joel Morris, a comedy writer. Joel has written prolifically for film, TV, and radio – his work includes Charlie Brooker's *Screenwipe* and the character Philomena Cunk on the series. He's the co-creator of the Ladybird Books for Grown-ups series, and his newest book, *Be Funny or Die*, is a serious look at the business of comedy. Where does it come from, how does it work, and why do we need it?

'I think the best thing about a good, funny book is that we're allowed to expect to enjoy it,' says Joel. 'If I know something is supposed to be funny, and I'm not enjoying it, ten pages in, I feel as though I'm allowed to put it down. With "serious" books, there's pressure to struggle on to the end. There's a lightness of heart and a joy that comes from brilliant comedy. And that's why it's worth holding out for the books that really, really make us laugh.'

Joel says that he grew up thinking there was a difference between 'real' books and the books he wanted to read. 'I'd get a book token for Christmas and my parents would try to persuade me to buy a "real" book with it, something serious. And I'd argue that if I wanted a "real" book, there were plenty of them at school. I wanted *The Tricksters' Handbook* or *The Usborne Spy's Guidebook* or anything with loads of drawings. The funniest book I ever read in my life – the one that made me think I would die laughing reading it – was the cartoonist Leo Baxendale's *Willie the Kid*. That experience, of laughing so hard, was magical. I loved anything with pictures. Comics count as reading. Graphic novels count as books. And I'd never tell my own child that those things aren't worth reading – anything that brings us that much joy is worth reading.'

Like me, Joel is neurodivergent, and he suspects that neurodivergent readers approach text in a different way, which might make comic books especially appealing to us. 'I don't always read in a focused, measured, paragraph-by-paragraph way,' he explains, 'and I found this especially tricky when I was younger. I think that, because I'm always searching for a dopamine hit, I'm always seeking out hidden rewards, panning for something that will make me laugh. Perhaps anything visual is especially rewarding for readers like us because we can usually find great jokes tucked away in the background.'

Joel also has an interesting theory about books being the perfect format for comedy. 'We don't necessarily expect to laugh when we read because we associate reading with quiet and being focused. We laugh when we're shocked or surprised – and the delicious surprise of finding something funny *in* a book is the surprise. For this reason, I think funny books feel more intimate and inclusive. The author doesn't need to hold anyone at arms' length to create more surprises, there's warmth. They can pull you in. And the funniest books work like sitcoms. I reread *Winnie-the-Pooh* every few years because it's a masterpiece in comic prose. It works because you can instantly identify every character clearly. And you revel in the moments when Eeyore does something especially misanthropic and Eeyoreish – in the way that you laugh when Monica vacuums her vacuum in a repeat of *Friends,* even though you've seen her do it before. It's familiar, comforting and reassuring.'

He believes that reading funny books has made him a much more confident all-round reader. 'Some of the best advice I ever got about reading came from a teacher at school, who said that if I wanted to understand the classics, and how writers like Austen and Dickens got to work, I should start by looking at parodies of their work. Because those are written by people who have studied the literary conventions – you need to understand the text to make those jokes. And when I could laugh at those jokes, I could understand the framework of the original text. Also, that was how I discovered that Austen and Dickens were *already* funny writers. I think school ruins reading for so many of us, in the way that PE ruins exercise for so many of us. The "big books" are daunting and we believe they're going to be dry, dusty, and serious before we open them. It's such a surprise, and a source of delight, when we realise that they're funny – and they're *good.* They weren't written to torment overwhelmed 14-year-olds, they're a genuine pleasure to read.'

So where should we look if we want to find a book that will make us laugh? 'I'm always surprised by how small the "humour" section is, even in the bigger bookshops,' says Joel. 'I like looking for annuals from junk shops and car boot sales. Things like the Giles cartoons, which are a way to travel back in time and remember what was in the news and what we were making fun of in the 80s. I love script books too. You can read an old Monty Python book and see the scripts that were never made into sketches, because they were too expensive or didn't work. And, then, there are the classics. Douglas Adams' Hitchhiker's books, *Diary of a Nobody* by George Grossmith, and *Three Men in a Boat* by Jerome K. Jerome. Most comic novels are quite short. You could read any one of those in a week, you'd have a wonderful time, and you'd have read a classic novel! But reading funny books is about reading for pleasure and it's all about your own enjoyment. And the more pleasure you get from books, the better you'll get at seeking it out. We all have peaks and dips in our reading habits. For the first time in years, I'm reading novels before bed instead of looking at my phone. I'm enjoying them enormously and sleeping so much better. But I'm becoming a reader who is getting so much from these books because I'm a reader of comic books, and graphic novels, and funny annuals.'

Like Joel, I think my love of funny books has shaped my relationship with reading, and life. Laughter makes me feel hopeful. I'm delighted when a daunting book takes me by surprise and gives me something to laugh at. But I think the greatest writers understand that life can be comic and tragic, and when we can find the funny side, we can always find the light. I've learned that I can read sad, serious books and allow painful emotions to come to the surface because I trust that I won't feel sad and serious for ever. We can always find solace in some literary silliness. And when real life is especially sharp, heavy, or lonely, funny books are filled with friends whose behaviour is soothingly consistent. If we're struggling with circumstances beyond our control, we can always rely on Kingsley Amis and Eeyore.

How books can make you feel funnier
- **Get serious about silliness** Sometimes, a book will make me laugh so hard that I'm giddy and I can't rationalise my response or even explain *why* I'm so amused. Children's picture books can put us back in touch with our craving for the ridiculous. I'd recommend *The Great Dog Bottom Swap* by Peter Bently and Mei Matsuoka to *anyone* who needs to be reminded of just how much fun we can have with a funny story.
- **Embrace the seriousness that comes with silliness** There's a fine line between comedy and tragedy, and we can gain so much from the books that don't shy away from this blend. *We All Want Impossible Things* by Catherine Newman is a

beautiful book about grief, death, and friendship, but Newman finds warmth, humour and absurdity in the darkest and most difficult situations. This doesn't make light of tragedy – it finds light beyond it.

• **Don't forget about comics**   We're never too old for pictures, and they can often enhance our reading experience. In the nineteenth century, most novels were illustrated. If you're struggling to connect with the text, pictures might bring the jokes to life. If I don't have an old *Beano* annual to hand, I might pick up Roz Chast's funny graphic memoir, *Can't We Talk About Something More Pleasant?*

• **If you're not laughing, move on**   Your sense of humour is innate. It may evolve over time, but you're allowed to trust your responses and look for a book you really enjoy. The question of what's funny is entirely subjective. It doesn't matter how many prizes a book has won or how many people have recommended it, if it doesn't make *you* laugh, you're welcome to put it down and look for something that does.

My favourite funny books

Cold Comfort Farm by Stella Gibbons
This has a classic set-up: poor orphaned Flora is sent to the middle of the countryside to live with her last remaining relatives, the Starkadders. But Flora is urbane, precocious, and on a mission to reinvent and update her cousins' lives. It's sparky, subversive and sharp-witted.

The Collected Dorothy Parker by Dorothy Parker
In Parker's world, comedy and tragedy are intertwined, and she ruthlessly skewers snobs, cads, and anyone who takes themselves too seriously – including herself.

***Love, Nina* by Nina Stibbe**

A collection of real letters that Nina wrote to her sister when she worked as a nanny for Mary-Kay Wilmers in the 80s, surrounded by literary Londoners. It doesn't matter how many times I return to this book, it always makes me laugh out loud – it's bitingly sharp, but tender too.

4
Read it and WEEP

"It is not often that someone comes along who is a true friend or a good writer. Charlotte was both"

E. B. White[1]

I'm crying as quietly as I can.

Holding my duvet over my head, I try to steady my breathing and calm myself. But I don't really want to feel better. I'm heartbroken. I don't think I've ever felt so sad. Somehow, it feels good to give into this feeling of total desolation. The sadness is bigger than I am, it contains me. It's an ocean, carrying me away. It's also like an ocean because everything around me is damp to the touch. I'm running out of dry space on my pillowcase. If I can stop crying for a second, I can creep out of my bedroom, get some tissues and wash my face. But this means walking past my parents' room and waking them up.

I'm supposed to be asleep. I don't know what time it is, but I think I might be the only person in the house who is awake. In a few hours, I'll have to get up for school. This wouldn't be the first time I've been told off for staying up all night reading, but it might be the first time I'm crying *before* I get told off. And how can I explain it? I know they'll say things like, 'It's only a book. It's not real' and 'Nobody died!'

But Charlotte died. Charlotte, the kindest, wisest, most generous friend a pig – or a young girl – could hope to meet. When I spent time with Charlotte, I felt as though I mattered. Real life, though, is a bit of a struggle.

I don't like school, even though I'm supposed to be clever. I'm good at the things Charlotte is good at – writing, spelling, learning new and interesting words – but that doesn't impress anyone. I'm lonely. But I never felt lonely when I was reading *Charlotte's Web*. If Charlotte could save Wilbur, she could save lonely girls too.

I don't know how to talk about how sad or scared I feel, but when I finished *Charlotte's Web*, the emotions came flooding out of me. And yet, I feel better. I feel hopeful. It's as though I've found a space for my sadness. It's moving through me, pure and forceful. Eventually, when I've not got any more tears left, I put the book under my wet pillow and sleep soundly.

In years to come – at 18, at 28, at 38 – I'll return to *Charlotte's Web* every time I need a big cry. Whenever I'm blindsided by sadness or grief, or a dark, difficult feeling I can't name, I'll pick up my tear-stained paperback and let everything out, with some help from a smart spider and a lovable pig. The last line has been etched into my heart for ever. And when I feel lonely or vulnerable or not good enough, I'll draw strength from it. No bully, past or present, can make me feel as though I'm worthless. All that matters is I try my very best to be a true friend and a good writer.

Super-sensitivity

Reading makes me happy. But sometimes, I want a book to make me feel really, really sad.

Crying is complicated. It's an emotional response that we can't always control. This can be especially true for some neurodivergent people, who report experiencing sensory processing sensitivity (SPS)[2] – a trait that 'reflects an increased sensitivity of the central nervous system and a deeper cognitive processing of physical, social and emotional stimuli'. Those of us with SPS often feel overwhelmed and struggle to deal with loud noises, bright lights, and strong smells. Many of us also report strong emotional reactivity and have a tendency towards tearfulness.

Sometimes, crying is nourishing and healing; sometimes it's really, really awkward. Sitting in the cinema at an early screening of *Lady Bird*, weeping silently as the friends either side of me cried into their popcorn – magical. Crying during a telling off at work or when I'm talking to a grumpy receptionist at my GP's surgery or because someone pushed past me in the supermarket queue feels less liberating. I'm easily moved to tears, and I tend to cry when I feel overwhelmed and out of control, which makes the situation feel worse. Crying over a beautiful book and allowing my feelings room to breathe means that my big emotions don't build up and reach the point where I feel unable to cope with them.

The rise of the 'weepy'

We've been crying over books for almost as long as we've been reading them. In the 18th century, the 'sentimental' novel was extremely popular. *Pamela* by Samuel Richardson is considered the first English novel. The titular heroine is a 15-year-old servant who writes letters about the relentless advances of her employer, which she tries to resist. Thematically, it hasn't aged well, but the response to *Pamela* shows that our appetite for a 'weepy' is timeless. It made readers cry then in the way that Colleen Hoover's books make readers cry today. It features people in relationships being badly treated and experiencing hope, despair, and confusion in their quest for everlasting love. Readers wept alongside the heroine. *Pamela* was a huge bestseller. After finishing another of Richardson's books, *Clarissa*, Lady Bradshaigh wrote, 'I verily believe I have shed a pint of tears.'[3] Readers were proud to sob, and there was a consensus that weeping over a story was proof of your 'finer feelings'. Indeed, to be moved to tears by a book was to show evidence of your empathy.

It's interesting that, as readers, we've always sought the sad. Even books for younger readers don't shy away from big emotions. The first book to make me weep was written for children, and it's a book about death. We have to understand that Wilbur is being raised to be killed, and Charlotte is trying to save him from that fate, even though her own demise is inevitable. Many readers report that reading *Charlotte's Web* forced them to think about death for the very first time. Lauren, 37, says ,'I don't know whether I knew about death before I read the book – and, even though it was incredibly sad, it made it seem less frightening. I *hated* the idea of it, but it was a very gentle way to come to terms with the fact that it would happen to everyone. It's a book about love and making the most of the time you have. Even when I was little, I thought that was the message. It's about doing what you can to make life count.'

Are we getting sadder?

In 2023, Gallup's global emotions report found that, across the world, we reached peak sadness in 2021, and there was an overall decline in our mental wellbeing.[4] This probably doesn't come as a surprise. The National Institute of Health published a report concluding that 'depression, anxiety, post-traumatic stress syndrome, psychological distress, and overall stress have been higher in the general population during the pandemic than before the pandemic.'[5]

The psychological impact of the Covid pandemic is still being measured, and many of us are also trying to understand the mental and emotional impact that it had on us. We were unable to do so many of the activities that we associate with maintaining our mental wellbeing – socialising, being with friends and family, going on holiday, maintaining a routine, even some forms of exercise. We lived through a sustained period of great uncertainty. We worried that the people we loved might die. Many of us binged on news and information – an activity that made us feel even sadder and more scared.

However, our emotional health was in decline before the pandemic. A 2018 Gallup poll found that we were all 'sadder, angrier and more fearful than ever before' and 2017 was a record year for misery.[6] It seems strange to suggest that, with all this going on, we might want to invite even more sadness into our lives by choosing to read books that make us cry. However, there's a logic to finding a story that matches your mood. Most of us tend to try to push sadness away. It's a complicated feeling and can bring up fear, insecurity, and vulnerability. We worry that it's going to swamp us. Perhaps worst of all, it's a lonely feeling. Sadness isolates us. And that's where books come in.

Andrea

In 2019, my friend Andrea died of a rare liver condition called autoimmune hepatitis. She'd been in hospital for weeks, and I'd hoped and believed that she would make a recovery.

We'd bonded through books. We were both members of the Jilly Cooper Book Club. Andrea was a reader – she was smart and serious, but she had a tremendous capacity for fun. She was the mother of two little boys, and was an enormously talented professional – a dreamer *and* a doer. She made things happen. She made the world beautiful.

After Andrea's death, I struggled to access my sadness. I knew grief was coming for me. I *wanted* it to come. But I didn't know where to begin or how to invite it in. Whenever I tried to think about my beautiful friend, her family, the life she'd left behind, I couldn't comprehend the enormity of it. Our friendship was made of nothing, and everything. Changing room selfies sent on WhatsApp. Quiet, clever jokes and references about everything from ancient classics to Jilly's wildest sex scenes. I simply couldn't understand that I could no longer message her about haircuts, trying to buy a house, or my attempts to read A. S. Byatt. On our 'Jillies' group chat, we'd all revealed that we'd more or less given up googling things because Andrea always had the answers. What could I do? I couldn't write to her and say, 'This feels wrong. I should be crying. I want to cry. But the air feels too thick, and I feel too numb. If I can find a way to cry for you, that means you're gone, and I simply can't accept that.'

But she had a message for me. She led me back to the bookshelf and told me the answers were there.

Reading put me in touch with the universal. Grief is strange for everyone. I didn't need to experience it gracefully or gratefully. For hundreds and thousands of years, writers have explored it, attempting to understand something that doesn't make any sense. And I found enormous comfort in the fact that I could read about death in fiction and grieve for imaginary characters, so my real-life response to grief might not be strange.

Still, sometimes I felt guilty and confused. It was hard to shake the idea that there must be some kind of grief scale. I worried that my relationship with Andrea wasn't 'enough' to justify the space her death took up in my mind. Andrea and I could have been closer. I could have been a better friend, a more present friend. And she had plenty of much closer friends in her life, as well as a loving and supportive family. (I still think about her family often and their generosity – and the way they invited us to celebrate and commemorate Andrea's life with them, even though the weight of their grief must have been too large to comprehend.)

In 1989, Dr Kenneth J. Doka coined the term 'disenfranchised grief'. This describes a grief that might not be viewed as a significant loss by those around you. 'Grief is a reaction to a loss, not just a reaction to a death,' Doka explained to NPR.[7]

Reading through grief

One of the hardest aspects of grief and loss might be asking for what we need when we don't really understand how other people can support us with what we're going through. It's even harder when we don't feel that we're entitled to that support and scared that our requests for help won't be met with sympathy and understanding. Reading through grief made me feel comforted and connected because it made me realise that no loss was too big or too small for someone to document. If an author had been generous enough to share a sadness on the page, I felt grateful and able to see that sadness as an infinite pool, big enough to hold as many readers as it needed to.

When we talk about grief, we tend to focus on it as an individual experience. But Andrea was a beloved member of a large gang of friends and grief is something we went through as a group. In all honesty, I think that made it harder for me. When Andrea went into hospital, the group rallied round. We organised care packages, rotas, and visits. We wanted to show her how loved she was, and we all came together to do so. There was a sense that, as a friendship unit, we were greater than the sum of our parts. We energised one another and our love was multiplied. We were messaging one another every few minutes, plotting, planning, and transferring money to one another for posh bath oil and pyjamas. There was always news to share. I remember a day when Andrea had responded well to some initial treatment and we cautiously alluded to a time when she might be well enough to leave the hospital. We'd all come together and celebrate. We'd never stop celebrating because this awful, frightening experience must be bringing us closer and making us stronger.

But when Andrea died, I didn't know how to bring my grief to the group. It didn't seem right to speak about *my* sadness when it was a *shared* sadness. Other people in the group were closer to Andrea. They had known her for longer. I wished I had more memories of her. And I felt guilty and ashamed of not being more of a comfort and support to my friends. I didn't know what to say or how to be.

But books remained our shared language. When it was difficult to speak directly, we still shared reading lists and recommendations. We read Craig Brown's book, *Ma'am, Darling: 99 Glimpses of Princess Margaret*, and we found things to laugh at and things to weep over. We were even able to give vent to our feelings through some of our favourite Jilly Cooper novels. I reread one of her later books, in which a beloved character dies, and my sadness took on a whole new dimension, finding a form of release. And my reading friends gave me space to speak about my imaginary grief. No one thought it was odd. And when I could talk about the pain of losing someone who only lived in my imagination, I was finding a way to talk about our friend too.

Like Charlotte the spider, Andrea was continually looking to see what she could do to have a positive impact on the world. She believed in the importance of words and the importance of friendships. Books brought our group together and they kept us together. When I felt isolated by loss, I was able to stay connected, through books.

Connection

I speak to Andrea often. When Jilly Cooper's latest novel, *Tackle!*, was published, I told her how much I enjoyed it, and how much I thought she would have enjoyed it – especially as it's about football, a sport that bemused us both. I think about the literary gossip I'd like to share with her, the books that would make her laugh, and I think about how generous and kind she always was about my writing. Several members of the Jilly Cooper Book Club have had their books published since she died, and I know Andrea is so proud of us and so excited for us.

This summer, we'll mark Andrea's five-year anniversary. This period is known as a lustrum – named after the 'lustration' or purification of the Roman people after the census was taken every five years. (When you're part of a group of Jilly Cooper fans, you might hear the word 'lustrum' and think of something else entirely.) I still struggle to find any meaning in Andrea's death, and sometimes I wonder whether I'm living in the wrong reality and there's another dimension in which she's still alive.

But grief can be like weather – sometimes the clouds part and the sky alters. Although every shift and sensation seems like it might last for ever, it always changes. On a sunny day – and there are sunny days – I think about how Andrea found herself, and the rest of us, through books. How reading made her passionate and curious, and she read for strength and comfort. I think of her when I need permission to feel sad, and when I need to open myself up to joy. Sometimes I ask her what she'd do next. Often, I ask her what she'd read next.

Grief and friendship in fiction

Reading about our greatest fears and accessing our deepest reserves of sadness can be deeply healing. However, books meet us all differently, during different periods of our lives. One person's healing novel may leave another reader feeling painfully raw. And this is why I put so much energy into avoiding Hanya Yanagihara's 2015 novel, *A Little Life*.

It's the story of four young men, living in New York. It focuses on the life and experiences of Jude St Francis, who was badly injured in an accident and struggles with emotional intimacy after experiencing horrific physical and emotional abuse as a child. I heard a lot about the novel before I read it. I was expecting a story of pain, brutality, and heartbreak. Some people told me it made them cry for a day. Others said it made them cry for a week. Perhaps it was the twenty-first century *Pamela*. But the more I heard, the more reluctant I was to read it. I believed that it was a good book. The reviews said it was excellent and I believed them. But I didn't think I could cope with that much grief or pain in one novel. I was happy to hear from the readers who told me that it moved them, but I decided I didn't need to read it and I wasn't going to.

Then my friend Becky, a keen reader, told me it was her favourite book of all time. Before I could say anything, she'd produced her copy and passed it to me. I couldn't bring myself to reject her kindness. She wanted me to love it as much as she did. I put it on my shelf and felt guilty every time I saw it. I'd have to give it back. Maybe I could pretend to read it.

Some months later, the guilt I felt about not reading it became slightly bigger than the fear I felt about reading it. I picked it up and braced for pain. It was enormous. I was going to be anxious and unhappy for *months*.

I loved *A Little Life*. It made me cry, although not for the reasons I was worried about. I thought it would be difficult to cope with the details of the abuse that Jude experiences, and the descriptions of the ways people are cruel to him. But it was the tenderness of the story that made me weep. I cried because it's a book about a man who inspires a deep, profound love in almost everyone he meets, yet never feels worthy of that love. I cried because it's a book about humans at their very best, as well as their very worst. I cried over the descriptions of generosity, hope, and collaboration, and the vulnerability we reveal when we hope, dream, and plan. *A Little Life* is about all the ways that life can be magical, as well as tragic.

Most important of all, crying my way through that book made me feel closer to Becky – and to my sister, who had been recommending it for years, and to every reviewer, blogger, You're Booked guest, and influencer who had talked about it. I believe the book affects every reader differently, and we're all absorbing the story through the lens of our own griefs and losses, but we're able to understand one another better as a result. And we can become more accepting of ourselves too. *A Little Life* has been read by over a million readers, so if you cried when you read it, you're in very good company. It doesn't matter how much darkness exists within us or how lonely we've felt, there are people reading with you, and they have felt those emotions too.

It's a heavy book – figuratively and literally – but the heavy feeling dissipated when I put the book down. I'd faced up to feelings I'd been scared to confront and I felt stronger for allowing myself to be so sad. I don't believe it's necessarily a book that everyone should read, but it will reach you when the time is right. Yanagihara's prose is painful in places – it's supposed to be – but that doesn't mean you're supposed to bear witness to Jude's trauma if you're struggling to process your own. If you're reading this and you still think this book might be too much for you, you're not obliged to read it. No matter how many friends tell you that you must because it's a masterpiece and they cried for a year and they're still crying.

Often, we can predict the books that are going to make us cry. But sometimes books touch us in ways that we can't foresee. I was excited about reading Glennon Doyle's memoir and essay collection, *Untamed*. I'm a fan of Doyle's writing because she explores her most complicated emotions with honesty and great courage. She writes about faith, ending a marriage, living in addiction recovery, trying to overcome the weight of expectations that have been placed on her, and the sense that women are 'supposed' to live in a certain way. These ideas resonated with me, and have done with hundreds of thousands other readers around the world. But my tears took me by surprise.

Towards the end of the book, Doyle writes about her daughter, Tish's, first soccer game. Doyle's wife, Abby Wambach, has suggested that Tish try out for a youth soccer team. Doyle has reservations. What if Tish doesn't have fun? What if she's not good at it? What if she feels left out? Nothing that she's done so far suggests that she might have an aptitude for it. What if it's safer not to try?

Doyle writes about being proved wrong by the sight of Tish, bright-eyed and running around on the pitch – an undeniable member of the team. Not the best, not the worst, but belonging to a whole that is greater than the sum of its parts. 'We are guided toward certain things: a pen and paper, a guitar, the forest in the backyard, a soccer ball, a spatula. The moment after we don't know what to do with ourselves is the moment we find ourselves,' writes Doyle.[8] And that was the point when I started crying, helplessly, just as I had at the end of *Charlotte's Web*. The book had touched me. It had prompted me to ask myself some questions. Like *A Little Life,* it had invited me to examine the feelings that I'd been scared to explore.

I didn't want to join a soccer team. I was pretty sure about that. But I craved what Tish had found – a feeling of *belonging*. Being part of a team, where no one is the best or the worst, but everyone is valued. Everyone has a job to do. I hadn't wanted to address, or even acknowledge, my own loneliness, but Doyle's book, and my reaction to it, told me that it was vital to do so. Still, as I was reading her words, I felt as though I was allowed to be vulnerable. I didn't feel lonely when she showed me the power of connection.

Breakthrough

My big cry led to a breakthrough. I realised that, while I need a lot of time alone, I need to balance this with some human connection. I have a lonely job. In many ways, writing suits me perfectly. Whenever I've worked in an office, I've felt overwhelmed by noise, people, meetings, and the fact that someone else oversees my schedule. But I missed feeling like a valued member of a team. I wanted to collaborate. I wanted to create a place I needed to go, where I wasn't continually alone, in my own head.

I'd been avoiding my craving for connection for all the reasons Doyle tries to put Tish off soccer. What if I tried something and I wasn't good at it, and people didn't like me? What if I tried to find a group to belong to, and felt lonelier than before? But Doyle's words made me realise that there is no way to avoid the difficult bit. I'd feel awkward, anxious, and far from perfect. But, if I tried, something better than perfection might be waiting for me on the other side. My tears had a message for me. I could keep crying or I could listen to it.

First, I approached my friend Lucy about some ideas I had and whether she'd be interested in writing something together. She was *very* keen. 'I'd love to collaborate and, if we get our heads together, I might be able to get out of mine for a bit,' she said. That was the easy bit.

Then, I did something I'd been putting off. I'd been curious about joining a local sober meet-up group, but I kept talking myself out of it. I was scared. What if no one spoke to me? What if everyone thought I was weird? What if everyone else had stories about waking up on cross-Channel ferries with Keith Richards and had no time for someone who'd quit drinking because it made her 'anxious and sad'?

I took a deep breath and went along to a session. It was ten minutes' walk away, and it lasted an hour. All I had to do was get through the hour. Ronnie, the founder, was – and is – one of the warmest, most welcoming people I've ever met. Everyone was different, yet everyone was the same. We were just a group of people trying our best and doing something difficult, together. All I had to bring was honesty and encouragement. I felt like part of a team.

I thought about what I was missing in my work. Was it possible to do something useful, with a social element? Could I bring back regular routine, collaboration, and conversation in a way that lit me up and made me feel excited – while avoiding the anxiety that comes with an office, the fluorescent lighting, and the electric eel of anxiety that rose up in my chest when someone crept behind me, put their hand on my shoulder and said, 'Quick chat?'

I saw a job advertisement for a part-time creative writing tutor and I thought it looked perfect. I loved the idea of spending time with students, asking them about what made them passionate, curious, and sharing some of the skills and ideas I'd picked up after all those hours alone with my laptop. And when I didn't get the job, I felt down for a couple of days. Then I decided to create my own course and build my dream job myself.

I've had the privilege of working with more than 50 students, and I've learned so much from them. Again, I've learned that we have nothing and everything in common, and so many of our biggest creative fears are universal. My own writing practice has become much more nourishing as a result. I can appreciate the time I spend by myself because I also appreciate the time I spend with this group of writers. When I wept over Glennon Doyle's words, I was able to acknowledge dreams and desires that I'd buried deep within me. I had no idea what I wanted, until I wept over a soccer game.

Books can help us to release our biggest and most painful emotions. Sometimes a story makes us cry and brings us closure.

We're able to release ourselves from something we can't let go of. And sometimes we cry and it marks a beginning. Sometimes our sadness might feel as big as an ocean. But when the right book helps us to release it, we can glimpse the shore.

How – and why – to have a good cry

• **Ease into it**   It's natural to fear negative emotions and to resist them. Also, if you're struggling with your mental health, you might find it difficult to cry. Suffering from depression can lead to feelings of flatness and emotional numbness.[9] And regardless of any other health conditions, most of us have trained ourselves to supress and resist tears. Don't worry if you *want* to weep, but you feel as though you've been bottling everything up for so long that you can't release your tears. Trust that it will take a bit of time and practise.

• **Be open to the unexpected**   I'm always catching myself 'crying for no reason', but there's *always* a reason. Sometimes a TV programme will catch me unawares and bring back an old memory or a complicated feeling that I haven't addressed. Sometimes my tears simply mean that I'm frustrated or very tired. Tears are a signal: when they catch us off guard, it's important to listen to them.

• **Try writing after reading**   If a book has moved you, sometimes a little bit of journaling can help you to unpick the complicated feelings it has brought up. I love the journaling practice from Julia Cameron's creativity course, *The Artist's Way*. Julia recommends writing morning pages – three pages of handwritten, stream of consciousness scribbling. You don't have to do this in the morning. You could try setting a timer for five minutes after reading and write down the words and phrases that come to you.

• **Give yourself time, space, and quiet**   It can be difficult for us to carve out time to be alone with our thoughts, and ourselves. But I find that, if a book has affected me, even five minutes of doing 'nothing' – being on my own and reflecting on how it has moved me – leaves me feeling emotionally stronger and more resilient for it, and I'm better at absorbing and using the lessons it has taught me.

Stories that make me cry

Tomorrow, and Tomorrow, and Tomorrow by Gabrielle Zevin

This story about friendship, love, and creative collaboration made me weep. Sadie and Sam meet as children and encounter each other as young adults. They bring the best out of each other and build a world together. Zevin's story is filled with moments of joy, happiness, and triumph, which means the elements of tragedy land extra hard. Ultimately, it's a story about how love makes us vulnerable, and why loving one another is still the best thing we can do. It's beautiful and heartbreaking in the best way.

An American Marriage by Tayari Jones

A powerful novel about a miscarriage of justice. Roy, newly married to Celestial, is wrongly accused of rape, and their marriage begins with Roy's incarceration. It's about racism in the USA and the bigotry that leads to a young man losing his freedom and his future, but it's also about the complexities of romantic relationships, compatibility, fidelity, how we lose ourselves in partnerships, and how we long to be seen. This won the Women's Prize for Fiction in 2019. Roy and Celestial are so brilliantly drawn, it's hard not to cry as the story reaches its quietly devastating conclusion.

Our Spoons Came from Woolworths by Barbara Comyns

This autobiographical novel tells the story of Sophia and her difficult marriage to Charles, an artist. The story begins with joy and humour – I thought I was going to be reading about bohemian living in the 30s – but it becomes heartbreaking as Sophia struggles with poverty, neglect, and emotional abuse from Charles. Sophia's voice is light, clear, and courageous, and her struggles earn her a happy ending. But this story of trying to sustain hope throughout hopeless times made me weep.

O Caledonia by Elspeth Barker

A sharp, witty, Gothic coming-of-age story that made me laugh and cry. This is about Janet – clever, prickly, and misunderstood. We know from the beginning that her story will end in tragedy. She frustrates and irritates her family, and alienates her teachers and caretakers with her enormous imagination, her sensory sensitivity, and her tendency to take things literally. This is a book about loneliness, and creating your own world when you don't always feel welcomed in the real one.

5
Read yourself SEXY

"You have as much right as a man to an orgasm and the way you reach it is your business"

Shirley Conran[1]

H ere are some of the very first things I heard about sex:

- it's how babies are made
- it's *bad,* in almost all circumstances
- it's something that men do to women.

It's alluded to in every single TV programme, advert, newspaper, and magazine. Sometimes they even mention it on the radio! But you're never supposed to acknowledge it or ask any questions about it, no matter how deeply confusing every headline is.

There's a list of mysterious things that people keep mentioning on the news. I'm terrified of, and curious about, AIDS, pornography, drag, homosexuality, the age of consent, paedophilia, perverts, condoms, the Pill, Viagra, libido, wet dreams, and something very weird I saw on *Eurotrash* about 'love eggs'.

Whenever I try to get any kind of answer out of anyone, they fob me off with fallopian tubes, ova, menstruation, hormones, cell walls, mitosis, meiosis, and babies, babies, babies. Sex, I'm told, is a 'fact of life'. It's just a lot of boring biology. But, for goodness' sake, don't *think* about it until you get married – to a man – or you're going straight to hell.

Sex education
I entered my teens at the very end of the 90s, which meant that if

I wanted to go online to find out anything about sex, I had to sit in the dining room, while the family computer announced that I was on the Internet. Or I could risk public humiliation in the library or school computer room – and I was convinced an alarm would go off as soon as I typed the letters 'se'.

Luckily, people have been having a lot of sex for a long time, and writing about it. Great sex, weird sex, joyful sex, and strange sex. There's one woman I credit with giving me my sex education – Jilly Cooper.

I'd encountered sex on the page before, but her books brought the facts of life to life. At school, a well-thumbed copy of *Rivals* was doing the rounds, and when it reached me, it changed me. It was full of women who wanted to have sex and were allowed to say so! Women who were a little bit like me. Some were clever and extremely ambitious. Some were self-conscious about their bodies. They fell in and out of lust and love. They had affairs and made mistakes. But in the Jillyverse, sex was entertainment, first and foremost. Good sex was supposed to be tender, fun, and exhilarating, but things could still go wrong. And while today's teen reader would be quick to point out that it's a world filled with misogyny, there are no conversations about consent, and no one ever wears a condom, those books liberated me and set me free from an enormous amount of anxiety and shame. Sophie Kinsella describes her experience of reading Jilly Cooper as 'utter, utter joy... and I loved that my parents would let me read those books in peace! I think they just thought, "It's just a book, it's fine."'[2]

Another book that had a great impact on the teen reader of the 90s is *Forever*. When I interviewed comedian Isy Suttie for You're Booked, she said, 'You just have to say "Ralph" and, if you know, you know. *Forever* was passed around in my class as a sort of forbidden book, which is weird, because there isn't anything about it that should be forbidden. It's a very sweet, straightforward story about a couple of teenagers deciding to have sex for the first time and falling in and out of love. It made the idea of sex less scary, maybe for millions of us.'[3] Elizabeth Day adds, 'The book I remember being passed around at school was *Forever*. So much to learn about Ralph! And French kissing! I went through a massive Judy Blume phase – she's a great writer, and she taught me an awful lot. Not just about sex and relationships, but about female friendship.'[4]

Fact and fantasy

Reading can be a crucial part of our sex education because it shows us that sex isn't separate – it's one of many important parts of our life. It's connected to everything else that we do, think, and feel.

Book sex can be serious, silly, or sensational, but it often comes with plenty of emotional truth and some essential life lessons. When I wrote my first novel, *Insatiable,* the story of a young woman who becomes involved with a sophisticated couple, I wanted to explore the contrasts between sexual freedom and emotional freedom. My intention was to write about desire and present sex scenes that felt wild, giddy, and fun to read – but also to think about what we need from sex and the parts that love, trust, and friendship play in a sexual relationship.

As a younger reader, I started to seek out sexy books and, even though I had no first-hand knowledge, I was quick to realise what felt real and what felt like pure fantasy. *Forever* is a great example of a novel that feels very close to an authentic teen experience. In the worlds of Jilly Cooper and Jackie Collins, there's plenty of glamorous embellishment and invention. I suspect even the least-experienced reader can guess that, for most people, sex doesn't involve naked tennis, helicopter rides, or ripping the Versace pantsuit you just bought on Rodeo Drive. What those details show us is that we can all have great sex if we cultivate a great imagination. And reading is the best way I know to strengthen and develop the imagination.

But surely we've all got better at talking about sex? We must be much more open-minded than we were in the 90s. We live in a post-*Fifty Shades of Grey* world. We have feminist porn, AI porn, and saucy audio apps, and *It's a Sin* and *Bridgerton*. We can watch anything we want, whenever we want. Our strangest sex questions are covered on *Naked Attraction* and Reddit. Is there still a place for sexy books and passing down our precious, tattered copies of Jilly Cooper novels?

Sex in the 21st century

There are several different stories we could tell about sex, the world, and ourselves.

On a bad day, things look bleak. At the beginning of 2023 – for context, three years after the outbreak of the coronavirus and lockdowns across the world – it was reported that Gen Z were having less sex than previous generations, and many were becoming part of a 'voluntary celibacy' movement.[5] In spring 2024, *Dazed* magazine declared, 'Rejoice! The sex recession is over!'[6] pointing to an eHarmony study that found 20 per cent of Gen Z respondents were having sex daily, and 61 per cent 'enjoy being "sexually adventurous" with a partner'. (Although, two weeks later, the *Daily Mail* claimed, 'Socially inept Gen Z is having less sex than ever!')[7]

According to Google, we're having less sex because of social media, an incel culture, poor body image, exacerbated by social media (especially in girls and women), screen time,[8] the lockdowns, social anxiety, *Love Island*,[9] living with our parents, working from home, streaming, gaming, drinking less, and watching more porn.[10] But is any of this true – and how much does it matter?

I talk to Danny, 55, who tells me that the post-Covid conversations about sex reminded him of growing up in the shadow of the AIDS crisis. 'I cannot stress enough how *deeply* frightened I felt about sex, in the 90s,' he explains. 'AIDS was a death sentence. Being a queer, closeted teenage boy was tough enough, but I really believed that sex would kill me – and a *lot* of my friends felt the same way, at the time – gay and straight. Some of us were having some sex, but the anxiety was off the chain. At the start of lockdown there seemed to be a lot of newspaper articles about being single, and being forced to be celibate, and what was going to happen to sex – and I thought *where were you, 30 odd years ago?* Things felt much more frightening then, and people seemed to have forgotten all about it.'

Alice, 24, echoes this. 'It's weird that we've been dubbed the asexual generation. I've got friends who have a lot of sex, who go to clubs and parties, and want to talk about it – and friends who have been with the same partner for years or just don't mention it much. Generally, I don't get a sense that we're doing anything radically different from our parents. Every generation has some kind of moral panic about sex.' However, she adds, 'I think one thing that has had a huge impact on us is the sheer volume of porn. I don't like watching it. Not because I'm prudish or squeamish, but because it's almost too much. It's totally visual and, for me, it doesn't stimulate any of the other senses that are so important to me when it comes to having good sex. I think it's addictive. I think it's ruined the sex lives of some of my friends.'

In 2022, *The Guardian* published a piece by writer Annie Lord entitled, 'What has growing up watching porn done to my brain – and my sex life'.[11] Lord writes, 'People act as if porn has created a world in which women's desires are placed in service of men's, when really it is an expression of that world.' She explains how her porn habit limited her own erotic imagination. 'Any masturbation unaccompanied by porn made it almost impossible to climax. I used to spend ages dreaming up long, complex scenarios about teachers telling me off or that guy who smoked out of the window of the block of flats opposite. But porn made all that easy: you didn't have to think at all because it was right there in front of you, screaming *yes, yes, yes...*'

The slow build

Like Lord, my earliest solo sexual explorations were inspired by the stories I'd tell myself. I'd read, and then read between the lines. After reading *Emma,* I had my own ideas about what happened between Emma and Mr Elton during their carriage ride, and I wrote my own secret sequels about Lydia and wicked Mr Wickham. At the time, my access to porn was limited. By the time I was able to watch as much as I wanted, I wasn't all that interested. I could see the general appeal but, as a sensory experience, it seemed to miss so much. When I *read* something sexy, though, the thrill of anticipation was delicious.

In *Riders,* Janey seduces Billy in the bluebells, slowly, after a long, drunken lunch. The eroticism of the scene is layered and immersive. As a reader, I can hear the blackbirds, smell the warm earth, and feel the scratch of bark and bracken against my bare skin. I get to be Janey, and Billy, and their director. When the key moment eventually arrives, it's especially thrilling because of the time it took to get there. In the porn I've watched, you get there in about 10 seconds. I'm sure there is delicious, sexy, slow-building, anticipatory porn, but a fair amount of it features cheap furniture and distractingly dramatic hair extensions.

First, it's important to point out that porn is a label used to describe a vast spectrum of material and it's not inherently bad or bad for us. Second, my preference for porn on the page is just that – a preference. Reading a sexy book isn't morally superior to watching a sexy movie. However, it's hard to look away from the research that shows high levels of porn use can lead to compulsive behaviour[12] and the widespread availability of violent porn is having a serious impact on children and teenagers.[13] Performer Mia Khalifa has spoken out about being financially exploited by the industry, saying porn producers 'trap women legally into contracts when they're vulnerable'.[14] To me, that's a powerful argument for reading your porn. The performers only exist in the imaginations of the author and the reader, and they can't be exploited or abused.

The Fifty Shades phenomenon

In 2012, an erotic novel became the bestselling paperback book of all time in the USA.[15] *Fifty Shades of Grey*, originally self-published in 2011, topped bestseller lists around the world. The critical reception was negative, with reviewers criticising the quality of the writing and the depiction of BDSM. People made jokes about the heroine, Ana, and her references to her 'inner goddess'. Officially, the book belonged to the 'dark romance' genre, but it was dubbed 'mommy porn'.

Fifty Shades of Grey wasn't just a bestseller, it was a cultural phenomenon. To me, it seemed shocking and thrilling that an erotic novel, written by a woman, and primarily read by women, was in the news almost every day. People had conversations about whether they'd dare to read it on the train. There were jokes about it on *Saturday Night Live*. The response to the book made me think we were all desperate to read about sex, sexuality, and desire. No matter what we thought of the story, the characters, or the quality of the writing, most of us were curious about E. L. James's erotic imagination and the effect it could have on our own. When the book became a punchline, I felt depressed. Women around the world had taken it into their hearts and so it was instantly dismissed.

Vicki, 40, says, 'I loved *Fifty Shades of Grey*. I know it's ridiculous, it's not without its flaws. I flew through it. To me, it was pure escapist fantasy, and when I was reading it, I couldn't think of anything else. I have an MA in 18-century romantic literature. I hate that I need to qualify my love of *Fifty Shades* by proving that I like smart, serious books, too, and I hate the idea that it's a guilty pleasure. We should never feel guilty about pleasure. But people were so mean about that book, and mean about the hundreds of thousands of us who were reading it. I think people should have been much more curious. Why did we love it so much? Of course Christian Grey would be a nightmare in real life, but why did we find him so appealing as a fictional character?'

Arguably one of the more legitimate critical responses to *Fifty Shades* is the concern about what it's contributing to the kink conversation. Christian Grey wants Ana Steele to be his submissive partner in a BDSM relationship, but Ana does not hold much power outside the relationship or seems to have much agency in any of her interactions. As Vicki says, the appeal of Christian Grey seems to exist purely in the imagination of the reader. I don't know anyone who would want what he offers from a real-life romantic partner. Maybe the way to interpret the success of *Fifty Shades* is to understand that we don't need to take our literary desires literally. Erotic fiction can provide us with a safe, fun form of escape, and some respite from everything that clamours for our attention. When we read, we can be anyone we want, *with* anyone we want, in a way that's completely immersive and completely safe.

Romantasy

I'm encouraged by the growth of a new genre with an escapist, erotic element – one that is treated with respect by readers and publishers. At the time of writing, the bestseller charts are dominated by 'romantasy' – novels set in alternative universes, filled with fairies, dragons, and magic, that also feature romantic storylines and, often, plenty of explicit sex scenes. BookTok (the digital corner of TikTok devoted to books and reading) is credited with fuelling the sales of romantasy books, and it shows what has changed since the publication of *Fifty Shades*.

Readers are openly celebrating their passions, and it's having a powerful effect. On BookTok, people are proud to love romantasy. Mel, 41, tells me, 'There's been a definite shift. I read the very first Sarah J. Maas book and loved it but, at the time, I was quite selective about who I'd recommend it to. Most of my friends are big readers, and we'd go through the Booker shortlist together, but I felt a bit weird about revealing my obsession with "sexy fairie" books. Now, everything has changed. Some of my snobbiest friends are asking for my romantasy recommendations and asking me where they should start.'

Mel believes BookTok has made all the difference. 'I don't post on TikTok, but I follow a lot of BookTok creators, and I think they're quietly changing the world with what they're reading. They have made it completely OK to read sexy fantasy books – in fact, they make it look cool and aspirational. And it feels as though the stories are becoming more inclusive too. I see more queer characters and more characters who aren't white – and I think that's definitely worth celebrating. This chimes with the words of BookTok creator Tasnim Geedi, who told CBC Radio, 'now that we're seeing a lot more diverse authors, a lot more female authors in the space, I think that's making it much more successful on TikTok, and also, like, the mass market in general.'[16]

It's heartening to hear that so many new readers are finding fiction that resonates with them – stories that are otherworldly, yet feel real in terms of representation. I think it's significant that these novels integrate the erotic with romantic and fantastical elements. Maybe romantasy is flourishing for the same reasons that caused *Fifty Shades* to soar? Perhaps we crave erotic stories that go beyond the bounds of reality – especially if we've ever been made to feel any shame, anxiety, or guilt about our body or our sexuality. Personally, I've never connected with porn because it's usually delivered to me without context. I'm turned on by Billy and Janie's storyline in *Riders* because I yearn alongside them. I was there when Janie slipped her dress over her head as she got dressed for the day, which makes it even more exciting for me when she slips it off again. These are the details that make it easy for me to fall into the story and focus on my own arousal without getting distracted.

But can escaping into sexy books enhance our 'real' sex life?

'We have to create a lot of allowances to tap into the parts of our desire that might feel shameful.'

To find out about the more positive effects of reading erotic fiction, I interviewed author and sex educator Ruby Rare. Ruby tells me, 'So much of reading and fantasy is about reconnecting with the aspect of play, through sex, desire, and bodies. A key message that we miss in terms of sex education and our sexual expectations is that play is vital. There can be an earnest seriousness when it comes to "performing" sex. Creating fantasy spaces and encouraging an imaginative approach can allow us to go much deeper, and into more vulnerable places.'

Ruby explains that reading erotica had a huge impact on her when she was a teenager, and now that she's 30, she's starting to rediscover it. 'I loved Jackie Collins – I still love Jackie Collins. Those are the books that I pick up when I want something titillating, but also soothing. The worlds she builds are so familiar to me – they're glamorous, comforting, kind of ridiculous – and hot!' She adds, 'But I also read loads of DIY things online. Fan fiction, but also loads of different self-published stories. More than porn, it allows me to tap into my own sexuality. It was a chance to dive into other people's smutty brains. Now, I've started intentionally reading stuff I wouldn't necessarily be drawn to in my daily life and discovering that it's really hot when it's part of someone else's storytelling.'

It's important to clarify that watching porn isn't inherently 'bad' and reading erotica isn't inherently 'good'. Ruby says that, for her, both are part of her sexual journey and both have had a positive impact on her. 'What's going on around body image generally can be very challenging and difficult. But mainstream porn sites were the first places where I saw other mixed race people, naked, who had bodies like mine. Seeing other people with brown nipples and brown vulvas and thinking, 'Wow, they look like me' was really nice. I came with curiosity, and I found some things that were really useful for me. But the visual overload can be intense.'

She adds that her experience with written erotica hasn't been entirely positive. 'I've also been listening to some erotic audiobooks – one was a mainstream, published one that had been recommended by a few friends. Quite soon after I started listening, the story went in a direction that made me feel *really* uncomfortable. It would have been useful to have had some more information. I don't want to know exactly what happens in a story, but it would have been good to have had some of those details clarified and outlined. So, at the moment, I'm data gathering, and reading from various sites online. Literotica is my favourite, but there are others. I'm interested in finding out what works for me in fiction, even if not necessarily in real life – and what I really want to avoid.'

So what's the best path for the curious but nervous reader? Ruby says, 'It's a bit of a Goldilocks situation, you have to try different things on and see what works for you. If you want to read sites with amateur submissions, you can find out what you really like before you start spending a lot of money! Crucially, you can let yourself enjoy something without feeling that you need to try it in real life.'

Ruby's point reminds me of one of my favourite sexy, scandalous novels – *Lace* and its iconic goldfish scene. I remember finding it thrilling on the page without having any urge to attempt to recreate the moment in real life. Also, it was *safe* to enjoy it. *Lace* was a bestselling book, beloved by a huge number of readers. There was a huge demand for that book. No one said to Shirley Conran, 'This is perverted and we can't publish it. You have a weird, shameful imagination.' Every sex scene I read that seemed out of the ordinary brought me release and relief. Even though I wanted to be alone with these books, I was never alone, in a broader sense. There were plenty of writers who were willing to explore the strange.

Ruby says, 'We have to create a lot of allowances to tap into the parts of our desire that maybe feel a bit more shameful. Especially those of us who are more feminine or have been raised as women.

Reading or engaging with written erotica can really help with that. It's all about finding a way to express our sexuality that is based around agency, and our own pleasure and exploration. A good example of that is the "ravishment" fantasy, or a non-consensual erotic scenario. This is not the same as sexual assault because it's happening in a fantasy space. There's so much danger tied up with real-life sex. We're taught that from an early age. It makes sense that we lean into that in fantasy spaces and give ourselves permission to enjoy it in a safe way.'

I think about one of my favourite 'sexy' books, *Les Liaisons Dangereuses*, which was assigned reading for my English Literature degree. I was expecting the novel to be quite dry, so I felt startled, and guilty, when I found myself enjoying Valmont's 'ravishment' of Cécile – a deliberate act of seduction and corruption, masterminded by the Marquise de Merteuil. Did it make me a bad feminist or a tool of the patriarchy?

Ruby has a theory about why that specific fantasy might be so appealing. 'We can think of it as an act of care. I was speaking at a conference about ravishment fantasies and I had a conversation with a woman who told me that she's so busy with work and her family, and she has to make so many decisions for herself and for other people, that her fantasy is not to have to make any more decisions and getting someone else to hold the reins.' While it's great to be able to do that with a trusted partner, perhaps reading erotica is a more accessible way to experience that level of care. When we read, we can submit entirely, and safely, to someone else's imagination and let them guide us.

According to Ruby, there's one more serious benefit we can all experience, if we want to start reading erotica. 'There's a difference between a shameful secret and something that's constantly private. I think it's important for us all to maintain private inner worlds, especially now, when there seems to be so much pressure on us all to publish the details of our lives and make ourselves available to everyone. We don't need our private thoughts and desires to be sources of shame, and it's good to get into the habit of creating and maintaining that headspace – a place that's just for us.'

This makes perfect sense. I love reading because it has helped me to find pleasure and joy when I'm by myself. If we have a great book to read, spending time alone with it feels like a positive choice. And if we have a great *sexy* book to read, we can reframe our experiences of sexuality and desire in an independent way. Reading for pleasure – *that* kind of pleasure – can strengthen our sense of sexual autonomy. It's a way to simultaneously experience desire and desirability without waiting for someone else to want us.

Getting between the covers

Maybe it's been for ever since a battered copy of *Forever* was in circulation in your school locker room. Perhaps you stopped reading sauce because you didn't love *Lace*, and the sexy fish? Or you'd love to read some serious smut but you need to find 20 spare minutes that you definitely don't have – and your Kindle charger. Here's how to get started…

• **Think about your favourite love stories, and love scenes** Maybe you were, like me, full of hormones and inventing your own secret filthy outtakes from Jane Austen novels. Or you've always wanted to know what really went on between Jane and Rochester. You could be a Wakefield twin, *literally* unable to choose between Todd Wilkins and Bruce Patman. Don't worry if you feel silly, self-conscious, or you can't get very far. If you start to use your imagination and try to explore the characters and story scenarios that have stayed with you, you'll begin to work out what you like, and what you're looking for.

• **Read in a way that makes you feel as comfortable as possible** You might discover that using an e-reader makes the experience seem more private. Or you might prefer listening to reading. There are so many different factors that might influence the way you experience these words. It's important to pay attention to what makes *you* feel connected and relaxed. There are no other rules here.

• **Making time is always difficult** You know your schedule, rhythms, and routines, and most of us feel as though there's not a spare second in the day. But this is an act of care, and I believe that if you can find 10 minutes for some regular relaxing (raunchy) reading, you'll want to keep finding time to do it. You'll feel confident, relaxed, and empowered. Personally, I've found that this habit makes me better at making decisions and upholding boundaries, which means I have more time for it. It's an unexpected benefit, but a very positive one.

• **Try to let go of any self-judgement** If you respond strongly to something, and you feel embarrassed about it, you're *definitely* not alone. But you don't have to tell anyone about it, unless you want to. Equally, as you read and explore, you might encounter material that's overwhelming, triggering, or difficult to process. Trust your instincts and stop reading as soon as you feel that something is too much. Nearly all traditionally published work should give you an outline of what you can expect, and if you don't mind spoilers, user reviews tend to be fairly explicit.

• **Be patient** This is a chance for you to explore, slowly – and to experience some delayed gratification, in a world where everything feels instant. It might take some time to connect with the right sexy story, but try to see this time as an opportunity. You're getting to know yourself, you're checking in with yourself, and you're developing an important private world. You're using your time and your imagination in a way that's just for you and, hopefully, you can start to savour it.

Your sexy reading list

Harriet by Jilly Cooper

If you'd like something a little gentler, Cooper's classic romance is subtly sexy, not quite as wild as some of her later work. Harriet is a shy, bookish girl studying at Cambridge, and she has a passionate fling with a glamorous actor, Simon. She gets pregnant and, in disgrace (it's the 60s) she flees to deepest Yorkshire to work as a nanny for brooding scriptwriter, Cory Erskine. The thing I love most about this book is that Harriet is credited with having an enormous sexual appetite, and her enthusiasm is one of her most endearing qualities – she doesn't need to be sophisticated or experienced.

Erotic Stories for Punjabi Widows by Balli Kaur Jaswal

A novel about sex that is fun, funny, compelling, and fiercely feminist. After leaving her community and embracing her independence, Nikki returns to her local temple to take a job as a creative writer and listen to the stories of local women. She's expecting to find that these women need a lot of guidance and encouragement, but they have *plenty* of stories to tell. This book isn't the most explicit one on the list, but it's a celebration of the erotic imagination, tending to your sexuality, and protecting your inner life.

The Stud by Jackie Collins

Another 60s classic, starring the fabulously named Fontaine Khaled, a wealthy married woman with many lovers, including the titular 'stud' and narrator, Tony. This is camp, giddy, horny fun. On publication, Barbara Cartland said it was 'filthy, disgusting, and unnecessary'. One of the first scenes involves an intimate encounter in a carpeted lift. The outdated attitudes held by the characters are much more shocking than the sex scenes, but this is still a sensational, saucy beach read.

Vox by Nicholson Baker

Two strangers meet on a chatline and, before long, the conversation has become intimate, and explicit. *Vox* is a very 90s novel – it's funny, sexy, and strange. The fantasies are layered, as Abby and Jim explore their desires together. I love this book because it's about the contrast between intimacy and distance, and because it taps into a key to fantasy – it gives its protagonists the chance to invent themselves and become exactly who they claim to be. Fantasy is a theme Baker keeps returning to. For further reading, you could try his novel *House of Holes*, a story of a sexual theme park in which visitors can experience their strangest and most specific fantasies.

Insatiable by Daisy Buchanan

Reader, please forgive me for including my own work but, as a fierce fan and student of sexy stories, it's not surprising that I wanted to write one of my own. Violet, 26, feels stuck. Her dream role at an art start-up is turning into another badly paid dead-end job. She's broken off her engagement and left the relationship that was crushing her – and she's lost all her friends in the process. When she meets Lottie, she's captivated, and Lottie and her husband, Simon, seem to hold the key to Violet's professional dreams, as well as some less orthodox fantasies. Violet is *thrilled* to become their plaything, but what will happen when they become tired of their new toy? Can Violet save herself?

6

Reading your RELATIVES

"All happy families are alike; each unhappy family is unhappy in its own way"

Leo Tolstoy[1]

"If you think you're enlightened, go spend a week with your family"

Ram Dass[2]

'Are you nearly finished?' Beth yawns. 'If you don't turn your light off soon, I'm telling Mum.'

'Shhh!' I growl. 'Go to sleep. I'll turn it off in a minute.'

It's a shame that Beth my sister isn't more like Beth in *Little Women* – endlessly patient, kind, and forgiving. I'd love a sister like that. But, together, we're more like Amy and Jo. We know exactly how to rile each other up and get a rise out of each other. And I wish she'd shut up and let me read because Amy has just burned Jo's book and this chapter is *electrifying*. I'm alive with fury and righteous indignation. I'm incandescent on Jo's behalf. But there's something strangely soothing and calming too. This is a story about how it really feels to have sisters.

My relationship with Beth is *exhausting*. We crave closeness, but we can't understand each other. We can't give each other what we want. I know I can be bossy, demanding, and manipulative, although I don't feel that way. I don't mean to be. She brings out the worst in me. I love her so much, but I find her infuriating. I don't understand her, but I don't know who I am without her either.

I'm aware of her tossing and turning as I stare at the blank space at the end of the chapter. And I feel relieved, even peaceful. I know why Amy burned Jo's book, and I understand exactly how

Jo felt when she was shaking her sister. Maybe I'm not a bad sister
and maybe Beth isn't bad either. Maybe having sisters is just *hard*.
Maybe it's always been hard.

Families, fiction, and freedom
Families are fascinating and I believe no two families are alike,
whether they're happy or unhappy. Families make great subjects
for novels because they're filled with characters who are forced to
spend time together despite their contrasts and clashes. But
spending time with fictional families can equip us with the tools
we need to understand our own, real ones.

When I first encountered Tolstoy's words, they seemed designed
to comfort moody teenagers. My family wasn't happy all the time,
but at least, according to Tolstoy, that made us unique. Unhappy
families seemed more interesting than happy ones.

If you're a reader with a complicated family, you're in good
company. Nancy Pearl, bestselling author and celebrated librarian,
has talked about how her complicated home life had a huge
influence on the reading habit that has defined her life. 'I was
deeply and fatally unhappy. It was painful to live in our house and
consequently I spent most of my childhood and adolescence at
the public library. The librarians at the Parkman Branch Library
found me books that revealed worlds beyond what I saw and
experienced every day… it's not too much of an exaggeration – if
it's one at all – to say that reading saved my life.'[3]

Reading can help us to understand our families, but it also
allows us to spend some time away from our families. As children,
we're continually supervised and overseen. I found reading
liberating because it was one of the first things I was allowed to
do alone. When I was a child, I was never allowed to run off by
myself in a shop or a café, but I was given free rein in the children's
section of my local library. Like Pearl, I realised the library was a
world filled with other worlds. It was a safe, calm space to explore
all kinds of new ideas and scenarios. For many of us, choosing

and reading a book gives us our very first experience of independence. We start to understand our families because we're able to start seeing who we are when we're apart from our families. We begin to realise that our families are fallible and we're shaped by them, but we don't need to be defined by them.

Reading has taught me that *no* two families are alike, whether they're real or fictional. But it has also shown me how to understand my own family of origin, through the families I've found on the page. Perhaps most importantly, I believe reading has made me a kinder, wiser sister and daughter. I'm not a mother, but getting to know a range of fictional mothers has made me feel much closer to my own. It's also helped me to make sense of my own complicated feelings about opting out of motherhood and being child-free.

Fiction is filled with mothers and maternal figures who are cast as monsters. It's easy to read *Pride and Prejudice* and laugh at Mrs Bennett's snobbery and vulgarity. It feels delicious to hate Mrs Wormwood from *Matilda* and to judge her for choosing looks over books. Novels remind us that we always expect so much from mothers, and women generally, on the page and in life. If we've ever felt alienated or misunderstood by the people who brought us into the world, we can always find a fellow lost child in a book. But books also remind us that our mothers are human. They're flawed, just as we are. When we read, we learn that no mother is perfect and it lets them and us off the hook. They don't have to be perfect and neither do we. And meeting so many 'monstrous' mothers in books has made me appreciate my own.

Sister stories

Because I'm the eldest of six girls, I've always sought out stories about sisters. For a long time it seemed easier to find families like mine in books than in real life. When I was growing up, most of the people I knew had one other sibling, occasionally two. Everywhere we went, we attracted attention – at least, that's the way it felt at the time – because there were so many of us. I was painfully self-conscious about the amount of space we took up as a unit. When we went to the supermarket, it was as though we were holding a small, badly organised parade. Everything had to be multiplied by six or divided by six, in the interests of fairness. Leftover cake would be cut up into mouthfuls of crumbs.

We seemed much more old-fashioned than the other families I knew. Together, we'd all go to church – for Catholic Mass – every single Sunday. We weren't allowed to watch soaps, get our ears pierced, or say 'Oh my God.' To me, in the 90s, doing these seemed like qualifications for coolness or, at least, social acceptability. Sometimes I secretly wondered whether we'd accidentally travelled in time and my family was supposed to be Victorian.

I didn't know any other real-life family that was like ours, but I found plenty when I read. *Little Women* was destined to be my favourite, even before I started reading it. Though I could identify with Amy and her selfishness, and Jo and her temper, I wanted to be more like Meg, who seemed very grown up. The message of *Little Women* seemed to be that life itself was hard, but your family was your sanctuary. And that, even though it is human to make mistakes, you should always try to be kinder, more patient, and more giving. I tried to make my sisters put on plays. I wished that someone like Laurie would move next door. When I caught scarlet fever, I imagined my sisters at my bedside, dabbing my brow with embroidered handkerchiefs and praying that I'd make it through the night. I was genuinely disappointed to discover that it could be treated with antibiotics.

The generation game

Our families have an impact on us, at the time and long after we've stopped living with them. We must work out who we are within these families and the families we create for ourselves. Some 30 years ago, my family seemed old-fashioned in terms of volume and values. Now, our set-up seems impossibly quaint. By the time my parents were 40, they had six children, aged between four and 12. I'm approaching my 40th birthday, I'm married without children, and at least half of my friends are child-free. Some have one or two children, but I don't know anyone with more than that. No one has a giant, bookish brood. No one has the time, space, income, or energy.

But nearly all my favourite books are about large families, siblings, and sisterhood. As well as *Little Women,* I read and loved *Pride and Prejudice, The Pursuit of Love,* and the Cazalet Chronicles. These are stories of belonging, connection, loyalty, and love. I've never stopped reading and returning to these stories – maybe I'm looking for answers. I'm part of a big family. I love nothing more than using my imagination and temporarily slotting into another big family. So why have I chosen not to have children? And where are the stories that celebrate marriage, partnership, and friendship as valid forms of building family?

Family in the 21st century

In the UK and USA, the birth rate is falling. In the USA, it dropped almost 23 per cent between 2007 and 2022.[4] In the UK, it's been falling steadily since 2010.[5] This has been attributed to a wide range of factors, including the rising costs of housing and childcare, and anxiety about the climate emergency.

My friend Tricia, 38, tells me that all the mothers she knows are struggling and she's had to change her own family plans. 'My daughter is an only child. But I've got two sisters – I'm in the middle – and I always assumed I'd have *at least* three kids. I've not consciously thought about it before, but I think I did want the big, storybook family. I loved those stories when I was little and, even then, I had Enid Blyton fantasises. I'd imagine having a little gang and sending them off on adventures. But, in all honesty, I don't know how anyone does it now, with two. In fact, I'm not sure that the people with two kids know how they're doing it.'

Tricia says that she still loves reading about families and she'd love to see authentic depictions of family life. 'I will *always* read things like *Pride and Prejudice* for escapism, and because it's a wonderful book. And there are definitely writers I enjoy who talk about their families in a relatable, funny way, like Gill Sims. But it would be great to see a wider range of families in fiction. I know so many women like me who feel guilty about only having one child – and I think that if we could see ourselves in more stories, it would really help to ease that guilt.'

Tricia's words have touched a nerve. I'll always love books about big families, but I'd love to find more books about women who live like me too. Sometimes, I feel guilty about the fact that I don't want to have children. One novel that quenched my anguish and eased my anxiety enormously was *Motherhood* by Sheila Heti. It's a thoughtful book about maternal ambivalence, and Heti treats this complex question seriously and with respect. It's a work of fiction about thinking and Heti touches on a kind of disenfranchised grief; her words eased some of my shame. 'There is a kind of sadness in not wanting the things that give so many other people their life's meaning,'[6] she writes. It's such a generous sentence, and I'm still so grateful for the release it has given me. It offers permission to want something different, and to feel strange about the wanting.

However, a great family story never stops reminding us that families aren't simply made up of mothers, fathers, and children. The world of P. G. Wodehouse is populated with aunts. *I Capture the Castle* by Dodie Smith is made remarkable by Topaz, a non-wicked stepmother, who is kind, pragmatic, beautiful – if inclined to embarrass her stepchildren with frequent nudity. Books often become especially interesting when a cousin is introduced. Although I tend to think of *The Pursuit of Love* as a story of siblings and sisters, Fanny, the narrator, is a cousin of the Radletts and being brought up by her Aunt Emily. This gives her a useful bit of distance in terms of observing her family and added poignancy to her craving to belong. My favourite complicated relationship in the Cazalet Chronicles is the tricky friendship between cousins Louise, Clary, and Polly. *Happy All the Time* by Laurie Colwin is a story about the close friendship between a pair of third cousins

– it's a book about finding and building a family beyond the confines of your biological family. Another 'family' story I adore, *Ballet Shoes* by Noel Streatfeild, does this, too. The story of three adopted sisters, the only blood relationship is between Great Uncle Matthew and Sylvia, his niece – but the former is absent for most of the novel, turning up on the penultimate page.

In his Tales of the City series, Armistead Maupin coined the term 'logical family' – as opposed to your biological family. This resonated with so many of his readers that he used it as the title of his memoir in 2017. Maupin's novels, originally a series of columns for the *San Francisco Chronicle*, were based on his experiences as a gay man living in San Francisco in the 70s. He wrote about not being accepted by his family of origin because of his sexuality, and about the families queer people built for themselves from among their friends. The Tales of the City series is one of my favourite family sagas. I love it for its honesty. To me, the characters' sibling relationships are just as authentic as Meg, Jo, Beth, and Amy's – they, too, can be distant, jealous, petty, and flaky, as well as loving, generous, and fun.

My friend Tom, 42, says, 'I'm an only child, but I've always loved reading about families, and I think books have taught me that family is a feeling. I would have *loved* a big brother. We could have built a treehouse or made a raft and sailed it down the river in the summer holidays! But I've seen friends with brothers and I think their childhoods were 80 per cent fighting, 20 per cent video games. Reading has probably had a bigger impact on my friendships. I do think of my closest friends as my chosen family, and I believe that reading has taught me to really pay attention to the way those connections feel and to understand what makes a great close friend. I've still not found anyone who wants to build a raft with me, but I live in hope!'

My earliest introduction to a family that was very different from mine came from a book. Jacqueline Wilson's *The Suitcase Kid*. It's about a girl whose world changes entirely when her parents separate, and she divides her time between them and their new households. It's a very funny, very sad, child's-eye view of divorce. Wilson sharply observes that the compensations offered to the main character – 'you'll get two Christmases!' – don't ever fully make up for her loss of stability and security. However, the book isn't a cautionary tale; it's written to comfort children and young people going through a specific life transition beyond their control.

Helen, a 34-year-old primary school teacher, tells me, '*The Suitcase Kid* is probably my favourite book. When I was 10, my parents went through an awful divorce. They were so bitter and angry. There was so much shouting, and there wasn't any money. My auntie found this book for me, and I honestly felt as though it had been written especially for me.

'I can't tell you just how much that meant, at a time when it felt as though there was absolutely *nothing* for me. I remember feeling so sad and so anxious, but whenever I read *The Suitcase Kid,* I felt calm and comforted. I still have the one my auntie gave me, even though it's so dog-eared that the pages have started falling out!'

Helen says that this book still has a big influence on her life, and her teaching. 'I make sure that I always have at least two spare copies on me, and I keep a bookshelf in my classroom that any pupil can use. There's loads of Jacqueline Wilson on there – I still love her. But I also look out for any middle-grade books – chapter books for kids who aren't quite teenagers – that talk about and celebrate families, and different ways to be. It's important for kids to see themselves and to see each other. Reading and sharing these stories with each other makes them kinder and more understanding. If one child is upset because of something happening at home and they're acting out, reading gives their classmates some insight into the situation. They want to help them.'

Helen's words are proof of something powerful. Books are kind, and they make us kinder. Perhaps, in some ways, they meet some of the needs that our families might fail to fulfil. We're asked to expect unreasonable things from our parents. A perfect parent is meant to be endlessly compassionate, patient, understanding, and consistent – a set of qualifications that no human being can meet every day. But stories can nurture and nourish the parts of us that our parents can't always reach.

Fictional families

Which fictional family would you most like to be part of? And which family would you struggle to endure a single dinner with?

As readers, we have the chance to experience infinite versions of family life and go through every iteration of comfort, chaos, horror, tenderness, and isolation. When we're feeling anxious and struggling with complicated emotions, we try to make sense of our feelings by examining their root cause. We look at our families and wonder what they could have done better or done differently. As we try to make sense of ourselves, we wonder how our families have shaped us, and reading about other families at their best and worst can give us some insight into this. When we know what we're missing - and what we're lucky we're missing – we can work out what we need and find positive ways to change.

In Barbara Trapido's novel *Brother of the More Famous Jack,* we meet the Goldmans. They're open-hearted, clever, messy bohemians, and Katherine, the protagonist, falls in love with them all, one by one, finding herself torn between two brothers. For me, the pleasure and joy of reading this book is that the reader can briefly become a Goldman, too, but I wonder whether being Katherine is more fun.

Her own biological family is limited. We meet her mother, who is chilly and suspicious of Katherine's academic ambitions. We fall for the Goldmans, as she does, and perhaps, also like her, we're drawn to them because their warmth and authenticity are unusual and notable. Katherine is with them but not of them. We see them through her eyes, not their own. She's a guest, and we know that guests tend to lead everyone else to better behaviour.

However, there's a fabulous exception to this in Charlotte Mendelson's novel *The Exhibitionist*. This is a black comedy about Ray – notable artist, narcissist, and poor host – when his wife, adult children, and extended family come to dance attendance on him and celebrate his much anticipated, decades-in-the-making art exhibition. His wife, Lucia, is too scared to tell him about her own success. His three children are respectively scared of him, appalled by him, and unhealthily close to him. And the rest of the members of his family are hoping to lay a claim to his squalid, but valuable, north London townhouse.

It's a story that satirises the way in which we all struggle to see our families as they are and the way in which our families warp us. If you've ever spent time with your family and felt as though you've briefly morphed into a different version of yourself, against your will, this book will make you feel seen and understood. It's a book about a Bad Dad. Ray, the villain, doesn't take any of his parental responsibilities on board (despite demanding constant tending from his wife and children), but the awful impact he has on the lives of his family is unignorable. This is a story about all the ways in which families are comic and tragic. *The Exhibitionist* is the perfect book to read if you're feeling emotionally bruised after a particularly challenging family Christmas.

'Family is really about being connected to the people you feel at home with. It doesn't have to be blood-related'

Writer Emma Gannon explored bold new territory in her debut novel, *Olive*, in which the protagonist is a child-free woman, finding joy and liberation in her decision to choose for herself rather than be swayed by society's expectations of her. I asked Emma about the way readers have responded to her novel, its original themes, and how she thinks stories about families will evolve to reflect the experiences of child-free women.

Emma says, 'When I looked at people with young families, my heart didn't skip a beat. I just saw what looked like a lot of hard work... and a lot of crying. I was more smitten with the idea of independence: living alone or with a partner, travelling, having a job I loved, family time, carving my own path – but nothing beyond that. Motherhood was never a dot on the horizon for me.'

She explains that, while she loves reading memoirs and non-fiction written by child-free women, she was struggling to find those stories in fiction. 'I always write the book I want to read. The only child-free fictional character I really remember from when I was growing up is Samantha Jones from *Sex and the City*! I still think about the line, "She threw a I-don't-have-a-baby shower to let everyone know she was fabulous." When I wrote *Olive*, I was definitely inspired by the four friends, sitting at a table, talking, in *SATC* and *Girls*.'

Emma believes that when we write about being child-free and read about child-free women, we can find ways to come together to celebrate our choices – and perhaps change the stereotype of what a child-free woman looks like. 'Books can really inspire people and help them feel less alone. *Eat Pray Love* was the first memoir I read with a child-free narrative when I was 18.'

Like Emma, I've been inspired, moved, and comforted by Elizabeth Gilbert's seminal memoir. In some ways, it's the inverse of a traditional love story, as it begins with Gilbert leaving a difficult marriage and walking away from the 'happily ever after' that women are still expected to strive for. Gilbert finds romance, but, as a reader, the love story that I was the most moved by was the way Gilbert found intimacy, connection, and family feeling wherever she went. I read it as a story of a woman who feels desperate loneliness when she's doing everything that's expected of her. But when she leaves, and walks alone, her life soon becomes full of warmth and people.

The success of *Eat Pray Love* (which has sold more than 12 million copies at the time of writing) makes me suspect that Emma and I are in good company – that we might be part of a vast group of people craving joyful stories about different definitions of family and alternative ways to live. Emma says, 'I was drawn to these themes for a while. Even before I knew I was going to write a novel about it, I was longing to write something. And I put out a call on social media, hoping to hear from other women who were child-free by choice. There was a big swell of responses and I realised there were so many ways to explore this idea. My favourite was a woman who said, "My friend's just had baby no. 5, and I'm still listening to 'Mambo No. 5'!" That was when I realised *Olive* needed to be a novel. I wanted to create a world where I could explore the topic from lots of different angles, without the need to centre myself.'

Emma is another lifelong Jacqueline Wilson fan and tells me that, when she was growing up, Wilson's work resonated with her. 'I love Jacqueline Wilson's family stories. *The Illustrated Mum, The Suitcase Kid, Girls in Love* – the unconventional family set-ups. Single mums, adoption, half-siblings. I was lucky enough to interview Jacqueline a few years ago and she said she just wanted children to feel less alone and know they don't need the perfect family to feel enough and be worthy of love. I think a lot of child-free women feel like they are sitting outside convention, so her books always make me feel warm and fuzzy.'

However, Emma believes that it's important to read about all kinds of women and all kinds of families. 'I love reading about women being honest about their lives and I don't need to have children to enjoy these books. Even though I'm child-free, I want to still understand this wonderful big magical incredible thing my friends and family are doing! I loved *Matrescence* by Lucy Jones, *Intimacies* by Lucy Caldwell, *Soldier Sailor* by Claire Kilroy, *My Wild and Sleepless Nights* by Clover Stroud, *A Life's Work* by Rachel Cusk.'

Like me, Emma comes from a fairly large family. I tell her that sometimes I struggle to understand why I crave the 'opposite' of what I was brought up in. She says, 'Maybe because I have such a large family, I don't have any fear that I'll be left alone in old age. I have nine nieces and nephews combined and that number might still increase. Some are as young as five, some are nearly 18, and my relationship with them is just the best. I love them so much. An auntie relationship is a special one – you can spoil them, treat them, listen to them, help them, nurture them, give advice, and then send them on their merry way again.'

We both agree that aunts in books could do with a bit of an image boost and maybe it's time for an aunt to be the main character. 'I do think aunts get a bad rap. Famously, the bad Aunt Petunia in the Harry Potter books. The ghastly aunts, Spiker and Sponge, in *James and the Giant Peach*. Miss Trunchbull is Miss Honey's horrible aunt in *Matilda*. Aunt March in *Little Women* isn't evil but definitely spiky. We definitely need a rebrand of "The Aunt" in fiction!'

She also believes we need more stories about chosen families. 'I believe the Latin roots of the word "familia" is about household, all being in a house or home. So, the way I see it, family is really about being connected to people you feel at home with. It doesn't have to be blood-related.'

Talking to Emma makes me think that, as readers, we'll never get tired of searching for stories about family, but the definition of 'family' needs to keep growing and evolving. And while reading can soothe us, bring us comfort, and help us to make sense of our families of origin, it also makes us feel connected and compassionate by giving us insights into family lives that are wholly unlike our own. I hope that more writers, like Emma, will embrace the theme of being child-free and write about women making choices and living unconventional lives. But as a woman without children, I'm also very grateful for the generous writers who share their experiences of motherhood, in fiction and in memoirs – perhaps especially because I'm not a mother myself. It's a privilege to learn more about that experience and to discover a different perspective on family life. Reading about women choosing motherhood makes me feel joyful about my own choices and grateful for the fact that, for so many of us, it *is* a choice. Reading has given me the tools to understand my family and to create my own family.

How I use books to understand my family better

Sharing books with my family brings me joy. I love asking them about what they like to read. When I talk with them about the stories they love, I find out more about who they are. And it's always fun to bond over a book and find common ground.

I don't have children of my own, so I love reading to my nieces and nephews, and asking them to read to me. It gives me a chance to find out what they're obsessed with, what makes them laugh, and what they're worried about.

Over the years, reading stories about different kinds of families has deepened my love and understanding of my own. The more I read, the more I realise that no family is perfect, and every member of every family has a full and complicated life of their own. Reading about families has taught me that there is no main character in a family, and everyone can benefit from more time, space, and understanding.

More books to help you make sense of your family
The Panic Years by Nell Frizzell

A generous and fascinating book that combines the personal with the sociological. Frizzell considers what it's like to be a cisgender woman nearing the end of her fertility window in the 21st century, and explores the ways in which it feels as though we have both more and less choice than ever. This book combines journalism and memoir. Frizzell is frank about her own complicated journey towards motherhood, and her feelings of ambivalence and uncertainty. She includes a wide range of voices, speaking to different people making difficult decisions. This book feels like a celebration of finding and creating families as an adult on one's own terms.

***Someone at a Distance* by Dorothy Whipple**

An exquisite domestic drama about a family being slowly torn apart by an interloper. Whipple's final novel, first published in 1953, is a subtle exploration of the emotional complexities of a very traditional family. It's about love and how protecting the people we love can have devastating consequences. It feels like a direct contradiction of Tolstoy's words. It's about a happy family, the Norths, who are vulnerable in ways they cannot begin to predict until a dangerous stranger arrives – and they discover their happiness is no match for this stranger's will. If your family feels more unhappily complicated than any other, this book will ease that feeling, and it might even make you feel more compassionate towards your trickiest relatives.

***Minor Disturbances at Grand Life Apartments* by Hema Sukumar**

I adored this story about a logical family of neighbours in Chennai, brought together by their frustrations with their biological family. Kamala misses her daughter, who is at university in the UK, and she knows that she's keeping a secret from her. She befriends Revathi, a woman in her early 30s who wishes her own mother would stop obsessing about getting her married off. Helped by Jason, a British chef who has emigrated to hide from heartbreak, they bond, helping one another to reconnect with their families of origin.

***The Mystery of Mercy Close* by Marian Keyes**

This story stars Helen, the youngest of the Walsh sisters. She appears in many of Keyes' novels, but this is the first time that she's allowed to tell her own story. The novel considers how our families define us, by telling us who we are – or, at least, who they think we are – and how we can come to understand ourselves when we feel lonely and misunderstood. (It may be helpful to know that this book contains a suicide storyline. I think Keyes writes about this subject with an enormous amount of empathy and sensitivity. Personally, I found her book to be deeply comforting, moving, and supportive. It's one that I'd reach for again during a dark time. However, I'd also advise caution and care if you're feeling vulnerable.)

7
Read yourself FREE

"I was in the grip of such a strong compulsion that I couldn't stop myself... it was inconceivable that I stay with the pain"

Marian Keyes[1]

"All addictions stem from this moment when we meet our edge and we just can't stand it"

Pema Chödrön[2]

It's a month before my 15th birthday. I'm in my local branch of Help the Aged, looking for something special. Obviously, every time I go into a charity shop or thrift store, I'm hoping to find a second-hand Chanel handbag reduced to 50 pence. But right now, my goals are vague. I'm simply seeking. I'm looking for a magical passport, a portal, a ticket to a whole new life for under a fiver. I read stories, I believe in magic, and I'm a huge fan of *Jem and the Holograms*. I know that this is how things begin. There must be a hat or a pair of earrings that will elevate me from awkward nerd to sophisticated woman. If I keep searching, I'll find the sacred totem that transforms everything.

My luck is in. I find it. It's not a hat, a handbag, or a pair of earrings – but a hot-pink hardback with a pair of bright green shoes on the cover. It's called *Rachel's Holiday*. It's about an Irish girl in New York, a story of parties, cocaine, and luxury rehab. The first few lines make me gasp. I can feel my whole body lighting up and tingling. 'I was a middle-class, convent-educated girl whose drug use was strictly recreational. And surely drug addicts were thinner?'[3]

At this point in my life, I haven't actually managed to get hold of any drugs yet. Drugs, according to all the newspapers, are terrifying, mysterious things that will kill you instantly. But I'm a middle-class Catholic girl who hates her body! I'm scared of drugs, but I'm much more scared of spending the rest of my life as a good girl, never having any adventures. I'm stuck in the middle of nowhere in sleepy Dorset, where my life is run by parents, teachers, and nuns, and nothing exciting ever happens to me.

All my life, I've been convinced that everyone else has been handed a manual that contains the secrets of the universe – and they've been reading theirs while I've been busy with the Malory Towers series. But what luck! I've found my manual. *Rachel's Holiday* is the book that will tell me what adulthood is all about.

I read it in two days, resenting everything that comes between me and it, like eating meals and sleeping. I get toothpaste in the book because I'm trying to read it when I'm brushing my teeth. Rachel seems to have my dream life – living in New York with her best friend, meeting fabulous people, and going to parties. But in other ways, Rachel's life is exactly like mine.

She never feels good enough. She's yearning for glamour and escape, and that yearning is getting her into trouble. She's desperate, restless, and secretly very sad. She has too many feelings. She's continually overwhelmed by guilt and shame – and she felt that long before she took any drugs. She's wary of everyone who is kind to her. And she nurses a suspicion that life might be easier and she might be more lovable if she weighed less. I read on. Rachel argues with her mother. 'I was getting the plummeting sensation so often that I felt sick. Guilt and shame mingled with anger and resentment.'[4] I gasp with recognition. That's exactly how I feel, most of the time. How can someone else *know?*

Rachel's Holiday is the grown-up guide book I'd been searching for. I don't so much read it as digest it, directly into my heart. But at almost 15, I'm too young to heed it's biggest messages. It's a cautionary tale, I think. A warning about what might happen if I go a little too far. *I* won't go too far, though. I'll have fun, but in moderation.

Over the next few years, I go too far whenever I have the opportunity.

Focusing on the feelings

When I first read *Rachel's Holiday*, my understanding of addiction was limited. The novel was the first story I'd ever read that suggested addiction was emotionally complex. It didn't focus on Rachel's drug of choice – cocaine – but on how she struggled with her biggest feelings. It was also revelatory to learn that Rachel didn't get 'cured' in rehab. She learned about better tools for dealing with her painful feelings, but those feelings didn't go away. As a teenage reader, I didn't have the life experience to fully appreciate or absorb the many lessons of this rich novel. However, it helped me to begin to broach some serious ideas. I could see that the key to understanding addiction may lie in focusing on the feelings rather than homing in on what you were addicted to.

At that time, the very end of the 90s, drugs were a media obsession and the tabloids were full of scare stories about overdoses and instant deaths. Leah Betts died in 1995, shortly after her 18th birthday.⁵ Her death was caused by water intoxication and hyponatremia, which led to swelling of her brain. But the news shouted about it being a 'drugs tragedy' and so the first thing I learned about Ecstasy was that it could kill you.

I was also intrigued and frightened by a different book – *Trainspotting*. Irvine Welsh's acclaimed novel was made into a film and *Trainspotting* posters and advertisements were everywhere. The impact of the film was so unignorable that I couldn't look away from it – and I was a child living in the countryside, with no access to the Internet. All I knew was that *Trainspotting* was cool and clever and my parents had forbidden me from ever watching it – and it was all about heroin. I did manage to secretly read a copy of *Junk* by Melvyn Burgess, the Carnegie Medal-winning book for young adults about teenage heroin addicts. The book became another tabloid totem, proof that the kids weren't all right. It was explicit and uncompromising in the way that it depicted the squalor of the lives of its protagonists. *Trainspotting* and *Junk* both followed the death of Kurt Cobain, who died by suicide in 1994, aged 27.[6] Cobain was a heroin user and the media were quick to conflate his death with his drug use.

Addiction was presented to the public as something both grimy and glamorous, and a problem exclusively linked to the use of illegal drugs. I added it to my secret list of mysterious things to be obsessively frightened of.

Rachel's Holiday was about drugs, but it humanised its addicted main character by showing me why she was drawn to drugs and what she was trying to escape from. I saw myself in Rachel. But it would take me a long time to understand that I was even more frightened of my own feelings than I was of hypothetical heroin.

In Keyes' novel, Rachel remembers being a child and bingeing on an Easter egg that she has stolen from her sister – an episode that leads to euphoria, then shame and remorse. 'This time I ate it all… the terror and shame returned, far, *far* worse than the last time.'[7] I was shocked. I'd stolen sweets from my sisters and those awful feelings still lived inside me – I was disgusted with myself for my greed and selfishness. But I loved Rachel and I responded with empathy, not judgement. Thanks to Keyes' words, I could begin to also forgive myself and let go of some of that disgust.

Fiction can be instrumental in helping us to grow, develop, and understand lands and lives that are wholly unlike our own. *Junk* and *Trainspotting* are both brilliant novels that are about class and privilege as much as they are about drugs. Burgess and Welsh focus on the kinds of protagonists who never usually get to be the main characters – smart, dark, funny people who aren't interested in broadcasting their vulnerability. Because of these books, I learned about lives that are wholly different from my own, and I believe that knowledge makes me a wiser, kinder human.

However, *Rachel's Holiday* slowly saved me by presenting a lovable protagonist who was so very like me that it forced me to start loving myself a little better. Johann Hari wrote, 'the opposite of addiction isn't sobriety; it is human connection'.[8] Feeling seen and understood is vital for our wellbeing. Some of the characters I meet in books make me feel entirely understood because they show me my own emotional state so clearly. Books can make us feel tended to, nourished, nurtured, and held. They never judge us. I've struggled with addiction, and if I hadn't stumbled on the stories that reflected my feelings, I would never have known that I was allowed to name my problems, let alone talk about them.

So how do stories make us feel better about wanting to feel better? And how do books help us to find connection after we've looked for it in all the wrong places?

Numbing

I believe that each of us has our own kryptonite – a drug of choice that makes everything seem brighter and more bearable for a short period of time. But sometimes we find ourselves reaching for our drug whenever life gets a little bit too hard. In the long run, the drug starts to make things harder rather than better. Some of us instinctively know our lines and limits. Some of us only discover what those limits are when we exceed them. During my darkest hours, I've crossed my lines over and over and stretched my self-esteem completely out of shape.

Food, my first drug of choice, was followed by alcohol and shopping. When I felt overwhelmed by anxiety, these three things offered distraction and numbing relief.

Perhaps you're nodding along and thinking, 'Me too' or even, 'I'm not exactly sure what the problem is here. Those aren't really drugs.' Most of us will overconsume at least one of them at some point – and by that I mean we'll use more than we need and experience regret. I've worked in offices where alcohol, food, and shopping seemed as significant as work itself. They were the subjects that punctuated the day. I'd compare hangovers with my colleagues, someone would go and buy a new top at lunchtime, or we'd consume cakes, crisps, and cookies when we were stressed or bored. I saw myself and my co-workers in books like *Bridget Jones's Diary* and *The Secret Dreamworld of a Shopaholic* by Sophie Kinsella. These were funny, relatable stories about women like us, struggling with Chardonnay, self-control, and credit card debt. 'I can't have just *spent* sixty quid without realising it, can I?' asks Becky Bloomwood, Kinsella's most celebrated heroine.⁹ The line could have been directly transcribed from a conversation I'd had with anyone I've worked with.

Throughout my 20s, I kept my three drugs on rotation. If I'd been overdoing it with the booze, I'd turn my attention to ASOS and buy yet more dresses I'd never wear. And when it came to food, I lived, literally, in a state of feast or famine – starving myself as punishment for the binges until hunger made me feel tense and tearful, then I'd binge again. I rationalised my behaviour. I drank too much and shopped too much, but didn't everyone? I usually managed to get to work and pay my rent on time. That meant I was fine.

But as I entered my 30s, I started to feel scared. My anxiety was becoming harder to manage. I was offered my dream job as an editor on a national newspaper and I quit after three months. I couldn't cope. I was crying continually and having panic attacks regularly. I started to see a therapist and we talked about my low levels of self-esteem and self-worth. I didn't want to talk about the pints of white wine, the shame, the feeling of not being able to trust myself to start drinking or eating because then I wouldn't be able to stop.

'Everyone else'

I didn't feel good in my body. I was continually on a diet and feeling guilty about it because only a bad feminist would hate the way she looked as much as I did. My 'diet' consisted of starving myself until about 3pm, then eating my way through the kitchen cupboards. The drinking was almost always social. I told myself I couldn't possibly have a problem. Everyone else I knew seemed to be overdoing it, too.

In my 20s, I'd experienced blackouts, put myself in strange situations, and woken up in unfamiliar places with unfamiliar people. Again, so had almost everyone else I knew, at least some of the time. We laughed it off and, if anyone expressed concerns for our safety, we shrugged and drank some more. At the time, I believed drinking was part of the general chaos of my life. It's a period when many of us experience practical and emotional insecurity. We're fledging and sometimes falling. We're trying to establish ourselves in the adult world, meeting new challenges, and learning from our mistakes. For many of us, binge drinking is normalised. How else are we meant to get through a bad first date or bond with brand new colleagues?

But my 30s were supposed to be different. I was married to someone I loved and trusted completely, work was going well, and I even had a little money. If I couldn't be happy with my lot, there was no hope for me. But bingeing was the only thing that would briefly silence the nameless dread. And my binge drinking usually led to binge eating. I was always hungry, hungover, tired, sad, anxious, and looking for something – anything – to take the edge off.

The shopping was another assault on my body. I could barely stand to look at myself in the mirror because of the weight I'd gained. At the time, I couldn't make myself understand that this was happening because I was abusing food. I thought I just needed to keep buying dresses until I found the one that would make me look better and feel better. I couldn't stop shopping for the woman I wanted to be when I grew up. Yet, every new purchase was a disappointment. Scrolling on the screen, I'd see phrases like, 'Selling fast' or 'Just one left' and soon I'd be typing in my card details, my heart pounding. It felt frightening. It felt like being in thrall to a drug that I didn't want to take.

During the day, I'd tell myself that I was a bon vivant – a woman living for pleasure and fun. But I'd wake up in the middle of the night feeling as though my heart was going to beat its way out of my body. If I'd been drinking, the anxiety was so overwhelming that I'd have to grip my pillow for support. The shame was visceral, chemical. I'd lie in the dark, crying quietly, asking myself a question that I didn't have an answer for: *'Bingeing makes me hate myself, so why can't I stop?'*

Searching for stories

In Laura McKowen's memoir, *We Are the Luckiest*, she suggests that we all have a problem with something. Many of us are drawn to overconsumption because we're struggling to accept ourselves: 'Everyone I knew was running, numbing, escaping from themselves and their lives somehow. Something big was amiss. This was bigger than alcohol or addiction. There was hiding and denying, everywhere. Why did we try so hard not to see this? Why were we so afraid to tell the truth?'[10]

McKowen's book helped me to realise that I didn't need to wait for an external force to make me change. I'd told myself that my bingeing wasn't a problem because I wasn't hurting anyone else, but I was hurting myself all the time. No one watching me from the outside would have said that I was 'out of control', but I knew that I wasn't enjoying my habits. In fact, every time I 'indulged', I felt miserable, worthless, and frightened. But I didn't feel capable of stopping either.

At first, I looked to addiction memoirs for proof that I didn't need to change my behaviour. I thought they would comfort me by showing me that I wasn't 'that bad' and bring me some reassuring context for my habits. After all, I wasn't crashing cars or burning down houses! I was just prone to a bit of hangxiety. But I saw some aspect of myself in every addiction story that I read and I started to realise something important. I wasn't the only one who was terrified of my feelings. I wasn't the only one who was struggling to administer the correct emotional medicine.

McKowen writes that, before she got sober, she looked to addiction stories too. 'My bookshelf was proof: [addiction] memoirs were stacked there like a small, private support group... in those voices and stories, I recognised something specific about myself.'[11]

I chased McKowen's book with *Quit Like a Woman* by Holly Whitaker. I loved the first chapter, in which Whitaker describes a friend turning up at her apartment with whisky, declaring that, after a break-up, she was going through an 'alcoholic phase'. 'I saw not only looks of relief but also ones of deep knowing – we'd all experienced something close enough to that to empathize,' writes Whitaker.[12] As I read that line, I breathed out, grateful for my own feelings of relief. Maybe I was just going through a phase. It would sort itself out, eventually.

Whitaker writes about the chemical composition of alcohol – ethanol – and considers exactly what it's doing to our body and our brain. 'You can't drink the same thing we fuel our cars with and expect a much different outcome... we drink-for-fun the same thing we use to make rocket fuel, house paint, antiseptics, solvents, perfumes and deodorants.'[13] This information made me feel furious. Addiction memoirs and stories were supposed to bring me comfort and solace. This was confronting. I didn't want to believe Whitaker, or her book. I just wanted to learn to moderate, take control and, most of all, feel happy.

I tried another book, *Glorious Rock Bottom* by Bryony Gordon. I'd read and loved Gordon's other books and articles about living with and managing mental illness. Even when she is writing about the messiest parts of her life, Gordon appears to be talented, glamorous, and successful but, she observes, 'I was two people in one, having to hide ever more shameful secrets under an increasingly impossible-to-maintain list of professional triumphs.'[14]

This was also confronting. In fact, it seemed to be a theme of every addiction book I read. Every author was a high achiever, chasing accolades and promotions, and proof of their value, constructing a shiny shell for the outside world to admire, yet living in terror that all the fear and darkness inside was going to burst through and shatter it. None of these books was just about drugs or alcohol. All of them were about women who felt as though they could never get life right, no matter how hard they tried. Talented, ambitious women, with very high standards for themselves. Women whose lives looked enviable, from the outside. Women I had a lot in common with.

Reading and reckoning

It took me a lot of reading, and *thinking,* before I started to join the dots. At one point, I threw *Quit Like a Woman* across the room. But I started to notice something important. Being with these books, and hearing these voices, made me feel safe, seen, and connected. The reading experience gave me everything I'd been seeking from my binges – pure *relief.* These stories forced me to pay attention to myself, and to treat myself with compassion and respect – because this is the way I felt about the women I was reading about.

My appetite for addiction memoirs was insatiable. I was binge *reading* now. But I noticed that reading always left me feeling better than it found me. When I was in the throes of a food or drink binge, it was as though a fog had descended and I had temporarily paused my life and checked out. But reading brought clarity. It made me feel sharp and present. I also noticed a distinct contrast between reading a book and scrolling on my phone. Particularly Instagram, which made me feel as though my chest was being scratched from the inside out. It engendered a restlessness, a hopelessness. An Instagram session seemed to trigger my excessive spending. It made me feel that I wasn't good enough and needed a different life – *but I could buy one.* However, books seemed to meet me where I was. Even if I wasn't ready to hear what books had to tell me, they never pushed me away. They touched me. They made me feel held.

Partying on the page

However, when I wasn't reading addiction memoirs, I was reading different drinking stories. I'd always loved boozy books, and tales of wild parties and celebrations. When I stopped drinking, I realised that I was a vicarious party girl. Every time I drank, I was hoping to experience a little of the bacchanalian magic that my literary heroes and heroines seemed to enjoy. In real life, I found parties stressful, overwhelming, and exhausting. Sometimes they were fun but, often, they made me feel insecure. Sober, I realised that, for me, the best part of a party was the morning after – waking up rested, with a clear head. (I still usually felt embarrassed about what I'd said and done, but the difference was that I could remember all of it with perfect clarity.)

However, a party in a book has a purpose. It's an imaginary playground in which everyone must meet with triumph and disaster, and readers can indulge in as much second-hand hedonism as they like without having to deal with any of the consequences. In *Octavia* by Jilly Cooper, the titular heroine turns up at a fusty drinks party in 'a short tunic in silver chain mail... I didn't wear anything underneath apart from a pair of flesh-coloured pants, which gave the impression I wasn't wearing anything at all.'[15] It's thrilling to experience Octavia's audacity. I can empathise with her insecurity – she wants to dazzle in an attention-grabbing dress because she worries that she can't hold anyone's attention on her own – but I can also experience the thrill of her exhibitionism without having to deal with disapproving neighbours, my body consciousness, or the cold.

Jilly Cooper's novels are filled with lunches, affairs, and extravagant parties. Someone pops a cork on almost every page. All Jean Rhys's heroines begin their adventures with a cocktail in a dark bar. P. G. Wodehouse and Kingsley Amis each made the poetry of the hangover a major part of their contribution to the literary canon.

When I was starting to reconsider my relationship with alcohol,

I read *Tales from the Colony Room*, Darren Coffield's oral history of one of the most infamous bars in Soho, London. It is an advertisement for excess. Why would I want to be sober and boring when I could be like Francis Bacon, drinking pints of champagne? My love of drinking was bound up with my love of books. Growing up, I had idolised Dorothy Parker, and alcohol was intrinsically linked with her legend. The idea of never drinking another Martini broke my heart. Partly because I loved smooth, icy vodka, and the sensation of numbness creeping down my throat and across my cheeks. But mostly because a Martini glass is a symbol. It means capital cities, style, and adventure.

Reading between the lines

When my relationship with alcohol, and myself, reached its nadir, I felt very lonely. I was convinced that a mythical group I'd created in my head called 'everyone else' could enjoy drinking in moderation. 'Everyone else' could, I was sure, drink a beer and feel as though they could be in an advert for that beer – relaxed, golden, with perfect body confidence. 'Everyone else' had 'normal' hangovers that consisted of headaches and mild nausea. They didn't feel as though they were sweating their soul out through their pores. Anxiety and addiction both lie to us. They isolate us. They tell us that if we have problems, it's because we *deserve* to have problems.

The more I read, the more I realised that there is no 'everyone else'; there's just us. Addiction memoirs deal with this directly, but there is truth in novels too. Authors tend to write about sad, scared, confused people courting disaster and learning from their mistakes. There aren't many characters in books who feel as though they could star in beer commercials. And alcohol is a source of inspiration. Not in the sense that we can all drink a pint of whisky and write like Hemingway but, in books, people turn to drink because they don't feel at peace with themselves. Just like in life.

Drinking might not be your thing. Maybe it's shopping. Or eating. Or gambling. Perhaps you read *The Secret Dreamworld of a Shopaholic* and felt a twinge of recognition as you observed Becky Bloomwood's impulsive tendencies. Maybe you felt an affinity with Mr Toad, from *The Wind in the Willows*. Mr Toad is friendly and kind, but his impulsivity and tendency to develop obsessions (horses and cars) means he is involved in several accidents and, eventually, sentenced to 20 years in prison. Mr Toad isn't a villain. His worst characteristic is his boastfulness – he's happy to describe himself as 'such a clever Toad'.[16] He's chastised for this, but I always read it as a sign of insecurity – an arrogance that belies a secret fear rather than excessive confidence.

Aren't we all frightened that we're going to be found inadequate? And aren't we always trying to protect ourselves? The more I read, the more evidence I've found that we all suffer from the same essential fear. It doesn't matter whether we're burying it with shopping, Chardonnay, or motor cars, the important thing is that we offer ourselves a little grace, understanding, and latitude. Rather than chastising ourselves for having a drug of choice, we need to start by understanding that this is a human – or, in the case of Mr Toad, amphibian – response to life's struggles. *What* we use is irrelevant. All that matters is we don't use it in a way that ultimately causes us to hurt ourselves.

Finding freedom

I didn't quit drinking overnight, but after reading and rereading these memoirs, I started to understand something vital. For a long time, I'd believed that going without alcohol would be a punishment for being 'bad' but, for me, a life without alcohol turned out to be a life with more freedom. Everyone's addiction story is unique. So was mine. The fact that it looked as though I was holding everything together didn't matter at all. The way I felt was the only important thing, and if alcohol made me feel out of control, anxious, and heartbroken, it didn't need to be in my life. Letting go of alcohol allowed me to reset my relationships with my other drugs of choice. I still had difficult days, but I was much calmer. I slept more deeply and I wasn't experiencing the anxiety spikes that usually accompanied my hangover. Put simply, I didn't have as many negative feelings to escape. I started to reach for stronger tools to help me through them when they arose. Books succeeded where booze had failed.

Now, I turn to books rather than alcohol when I'm struggling with my feelings. If I'm having a bad day, I'll go back to Bryony Gordon and Laura McKowen. Their beautiful words remind me that I'm not alone and, if I'm finding life hard, it's not a sign that I'm failing and I have nothing to be ashamed of. Reading about addiction hasn't just helped me to understand myself better, it's made me more appreciative of our shared humanity. Even if you don't have a complicated relationship with your drug of choice, I believe that reading an addiction memoir can boost everyone's empathy and give us all a huge, helpful insight into the minds of those around us who might be struggling. These are the stories that make us all more patient, kinder, and wiser.

'I was desperate to prove that I didn't have a problem'

I spoke to Catherine Gray, the author of one of my favourite memoirs, *The Unexpected Joy of Being Sober*, about the writers who reached her when she was getting sober. She said, 'I read *Dry* by Augusten Burroughs because I was desperate to prove to myself that I didn't have a problem with alcohol. I was expecting it to be a sensationalist story that I couldn't relate to. His life and his drinking would be nothing like mine, and I'd have evidence that I was fine and I didn't need to make any changes. I was quite chastened to discover that we were emotionally very similar. Even though I wasn't doing my drinking in New York or taking quite as many drugs as he did, I was startled to discover that we both felt sad and lost.'

I asked Gray about whether she read more or read differently in sobriety. She said, 'When I was little, I was a big reader. Every week, I maxed out my library card. I'm not sure I even consciously identified as a book lover, but reading felt as necessary as breathing. But when I started drinking in my teens, I stopped reading. Not consciously – I just replaced one habit with another.'

Now, Gray definitely identifies as a book lover, so how did she find her way back to reading? She tells me, 'As I stopped drinking, I drifted back to books, but it wasn't until I got pregnant that I focused on it. Everyone warned me that I would never read again, so I threw myself into reading as much as I could, before the baby came. I don't think my mental health has ever been better. I had at least three books on the go at any given time.'

Gray explains that she has to protect her relationship with books because they bring her so much solace. Reading doesn't just bring her pleasure and joy – for her, it's a key part of maintaining her mental health. 'Writing – and reading – for me, have a similar mental effect to going for a run or swim; they declutter the overcrowded room of my mind and throw back the curtains, letting some light in. They bring me the kind of space, clarity, and brightness that I was seeking from drinking.'

Like Gray, I've been paying attention to the way reading makes me feel. I've noticed how reading brings me home to my body and makes me feel safe within it. When I read, I am still, and my breathing is even. If the words are holding my attention, there's no room for my anxiety. I can't rush to escape myself, and I'm not overwhelmed by the impulse to binge. The books themselves have changed the way I speak to myself about the bingeing. They have helped me to see myself as a vulnerable, struggling human, and taught me that I have nothing to be ashamed of.

A different kind of holiday

I'm 38 years old and it's my anniversary. It's midsummer and exactly a year since I decided to stop drinking alcohol. I pick up *Rachel's Holiday* again. I don't know how many times I've read this book. Rachel feels like one of my oldest friends, but she teaches me something new every time I meet her.

This time, I notice that, in rehab, Rachel must learn how to feel her feelings again. Not just the sadness, shame, and anger that she's experiencing in the moment, but every single emotion she has bottled up and numbed with drugs and alcohol. She's horrified and frightened, but discovers that simply feeling makes her stronger. Slowly, she stops being so scared of herself.

And I no longer envy Rachel her New York life. I don't feel a pang of yearning for the wild parties any more. I feel grateful. I've spent a year learning not to fear my feelings. It's a work in progress. It's been exhilarating and awful, dark, light, euphoric, intense, and hilarious. It's not been boring. Sometimes I feel restless, and sometimes I struggle with guilt and shame, but I suspect that's all part of being human. I don't need to escape myself any more. I can always escape into stories when I need them.

How to read yourself free

- **Check in with yourself** If you respond strongly to something you're reading, sit with those feelings and let them rise to the surface. If you find yourself identifying emotionally with someone who is writing about addiction, the feelings are worth exploring. You don't need to have experienced life in the same way that they have for this to happen and be worthwhile doing.
- **Let go of shame** We all have secrets, regrets, and a little list of things we wish we'd never done. This is human – and reading memoirs, especially addiction memoirs, will show you just how human it is.
- **Believe in change** A good addiction memoir can be empowering. These aren't just stories about people reaching rock bottom, doing their worst – these are books about people discovering huge amounts of inner strength and recovering. These books are proof of all the good we're capable of and how we can change for the better.

Five books that make me feel connected

The Wind in the Willows by Kenneth Grahame

From the moment Mole says, 'Hang spring cleaning!' you'll know you're in the most comforting company. Emotionally speaking, this is surprisingly adult and human for a children's book about animals. It's about friendship, vulnerability, and forgiveness and it always makes me feel better.

The Unexpected Joy of the Ordinary by Catherine Gray

Through the lens of her own sobriety, Gray explores why we all have such great expectations for our pleasure, happiness, and wellbeing, and invites us to embark on a reset. This is honest, generous, funny, and life affirming, and it helped me to understand how appreciating the good is a vital part of staying mentally strong.

Glorious Rock Bottom by Bryony Gordon

A beautiful and uncompromising memoir in which Gordon explores the link between her own alcoholism and mental illness and invites us to be more honest with ourselves. Gordon's greatest gift is that she can prompt readers to free themselves from their own shame and judgement. She's a generous writer, and incredibly funny.

Rachel's Holiday by Marian Keyes

As the novel begins, Rachel tells us that there has been a terrible mistake. She wakes up in hospital, having her stomach pumped, and she's about to be shipped off to rehab. She's *fine,* she's not an addict, everyone is overreacting – but she likes the idea of rehab. She might meet celebrities. There will probably be a spa. Alongside Rachel, we learn that she *is* an addict, but she can get better as soon as she learns to understand and forgive herself. This book is resonant, relatable, and hugely lovable.

The Secret Dreamworld of a Shopaholic by **Sophie Kinsella**

Financial journalist Becky Bloomwood is in debt and in denial. When she's trying to escape her money worries, she goes shopping. She believes that, as soon as she finds the perfect scarf, coat, or cardigan, she'll find the power to solve all her problems. But Becky is already capable of so much more than she knows – she's brave, she's loyal, and she can change her life by harnessing these qualities and using them wisely. This book is a real, funny, forgiving friend.

8

Read yourself ROMANTIC

"Perhaps it is the loving that counts, not the being loved in return"

Dodie Smith[1]

My own love story is a literary one.

Dale smiles nervously and hands me a hard, rectangular package, about the size of my hand. 'Happy Christmas!'

I gasp, theatrically. 'It's… a car?' I tear at the wrapping paper – white, decorated with silver stars. Inside, there's a very plain book. It might have been royal blue once, but the cover has faded. The binding is slightly loose and fraying. It smells soft and sweet, faintly powdery. All the information I need is written on the spine: 'THE PURSUIT OF LOVE   NANCY MITFORD'.

My jaw drops. 'You didn't!' Glancing at the imprint page, I spot something significant. 'This edition first published by Hamish Hamilton in 1945.' I'm speechless.

'Do you like it? Are you surprised?' He looks at me hopefully. I throw my arms around him.

'It's the best surprise ever,' I reply, and I mean it.

When I met my husband for the very first time, he also came bearing a book. It was one of Jonathan Ames's essay collections. Our first date happened on the day after my birthday, so he wanted to bring me a gift. And he paid me a very generous compliment. He told me that Ames is one of his favourite writers and he said that reading some of my work online had reminded him of the Ames book. However, I can't pretend otherwise, I was *slightly* perturbed by his choice. Before Dale had said a word to me, he handed me a book emblazoned with the words '*I Love You More Than You Know*'.

Dale and I met online, on what used to be Twitter, and we

bonded over books. We are both writers and readers. I am a big believer in John Waters' maxim, 'If you go home with somebody and they don't have books, don't fuck 'em!'[2] However, I'd been burned romantically by book lovers before. Admittedly, this was my fault. I am happy to read anything recommended to me and some of my exes widened my literary horizons. To impress various bad boyfriends, I read a lot of good books – most of Martin Amis, a lot of Murakami, the poetry of John Donne, a little Bukowski, some Irvine Welsh, and the autobiography of former Hull City midfielder Dean Windass.

I regret some of the relationships, but I don't regret any of the reading. However, I found it much harder to get my partners to take an interest in what *I* liked to read. Until I met Dale. He treated our love of reading as a shared language, not a competitive sport.

On our third date, he showed me photos he'd taken after spending the afternoon in a rare books shop, filled with beautiful editions of old P. G. Wodehouse novels. So I opened my handbag and showed him that I'd been carrying around a well-thumbed edition of *The Indiscretions of Archie*. It all seemed too good to be true. I was suspicious, used to men who made me feel as though their choices were the best choices and mine were a little ridiculous.

I was falling hard and it was frightening. For me, the start of a new relationship was usually accompanied by anxiety, insecurity, and a dramatically reduced appetite. But I just wanted to be around Dale all the time, talking about books. What was happening?

It was time to go nuclear. I lent him one of the darkest, weirdest, funniest books I could think of: *Good Behaviour* by Molly Keane. If he said, 'What *was* that?' or 'I couldn't finish it!' I could pretend that we weren't meant to be and I'd have an excuse to run away. But if he loved it, we might have been written in the stars.

Of *course* he loved it.

When we talk about *why* we should all read, we point to the facts. We're improving brain function, brain connectivity, and memory.[3] We're increasing the odds that we'll be able to impress our family by knowing the answer to a question on *University Challenge*. But we rarely touch on the way that reading shapes our inner worlds. Reading for pleasure is such a private, intimate act. It requires a suspension of self. When we recommend books, we fall back on dry, dusty phrases. It's easy to say, 'Read this – it's a real page-turner' or even, 'This changed the way I think.' We don't say, 'This changed the way I feel.'

Every time I begin a new book, I'm hoping to fall in love. I want to experience limerence – an intense infatuation with a story and its characters. My favourite books don't make me feel smart, they make me briefly stupid, as though a spell has been cast on me and I'm completely willing to submit to it. The best books convince me that something imaginary is entirely true. I want to believe.

So sharing a favourite book is one of the most intimate things we can do. When we give a story we love to a person we love, we're saying, 'This altered me. This made me vulnerable. This triggered intense bodily sensations that I'm still not sure how to describe. I took this to bed with me. And I hope you'll know how I feel and that you'll experience some of these big feelings with me.' Of course, there will be digressions and debates in any literary love story. There may be times when one of you decides to read the complete works of Nabokov and the other decides to reread the complete works of Jeffrey Archer. One of you may hit a reading drought. One of you may donate old books to charity shops, only to discover that your partner keeps buying them back.

But during the 2020 lockdown, at a time when many of us were desperately searching for new ways to feel connected to our old partners as we faced the prospect of spending weeks and months with only each other for company, I fell in love with Dale all over again when he picked up *I Capture the Castle* for the very first time. Not just because there's something very hot about a heterosexual man in his late 40s who has the confidence and curiosity to try a book beloved by teenage girls. It's about romance, heartbreak and longing, and big emotions. It's a book that lives in my heart. I've read and reread it so many times that it's woven into me. I ached for Cassandra's experience of romantic love long before I had any first-hand knowledge of it. Nearly everything I understand about relationships is built from books. Love stories show us how to hope and what to dream about.

Why do we love love?

The way we tell our love stories keeps growing and evolving, but our appetite for the stories themselves remains constant. The oldest 'love story' is thought to be 'Istanbul 2461', the reference number archivists have given to an erotic love poem told from the perspective of a female speaker, addressed to Shu-Sin, king of the Neo-Sumerian Empire (it is also known as 'Bridegroom, spend the night in our house till dawn').[4]

Consider the enduring popularity of *Romeo and Juliet*. Shakespeare's play, based on a 15th-century novella by Matteo Bandello, is still regularly watched and performed *more than 600 years later*. A 2016 YouGov survey found that it was the most popular Shakespeare drama, with 51 per cent of British respondents having read it or seen it performed.[5]

I'd argue that pretty much every single love story we've ever read owes something to *Romeo and Juliet*, whether it's about doomed, tragic love or its opposite. Gail Kern Paster, a Shakespeare scholar and former director of the Folger Shakespeare library, writes that it's often the first Shakespeare work – and the first love story – that we're taught at school, 'on the grounds of its obvious relevance to the emotional and social concerns of young people'.[6] It is about teenagers, so it's appealing to teenagers.

When I was in a classroom filled with intense, hormonal young women, all of us longing to know how it really felt to be in love, we all tacitly agreed that nothing could possibly be more romantic than marrying someone in secret, then dying to honour your forbidden love. We were primed for *Jane Eyre*, another thrilling story about a love that seemed difficult and doomed. Fortunately, we were given Jane Austen too. *Pride and Prejudice* and *Emma* showed us that romantic misunderstandings could be funny as well as fatal.

Romance writing has always had a mixed reputation. We know that there's some literary snobbery when it comes to love stories. Until the end of the 20th century, critics were quick to dismiss anything written by women – especially if it was about women and read, primarily, by women – and very few people were able to call them out for it. But romantic books have always enjoyed enormous popularity, regardless of critical trends. Collectively, we have long had a huge appetite for love stories, as evidenced by the millions of books sold by Georgette Heyer and Barbara Cartland. And we still do – in 2023, data showed that sales of romance novels and saga fiction had risen by 110 per cent in three years.[7] So what makes romance so magical?

Katie, 35, tells me that she thinks the romance writers of the past were better than their more respected contemporaries at creating characters with depth and inner lives. 'I don't need to read a book about people who are exactly like me, but it does seem that in a lot of classic literature written by men, there are hardly any women, and no one really gives them anything to do. I think Jane Austen was the first novelist I really loved because every single character seemed to have some genuine dimension. What people were doing was informed by what people were thinking, which is lifelike to me.'

Katie reminds me that Austen was writing about money and its impact on relationships. 'It wasn't lost on me that love and marriage *wasn't* a frivolous, girly interest at the time she was writing. It was a serious, economic concern. Marrying for love was a luxury, in a way. It meant you had a chance of happiness – at a time when very few women had any autonomy and could make any independent choices.'

Hopefully, most of us can now pursue happiness in all sorts of ways without waiting for Mr Right or Mr Darcy, so why do love stories still appeal to us? Katie says, 'I suppose it's illogical, like love itself. I think that in contemporary love stories we maybe see more examples of chance, accident, and coincidence – a kind of real-world magic that we want to believe in.'

Becki, 21, describes herself as a 'romance addict' but that that comes with complications. 'I read, and love, a lot of "straight" romance, but do think quite a lot of it fails the Bechdel test! It's full of straight, white people, full of women obsessing about men. But I think that, in the last five years, the stories have become a bit broader – and a good romance is great because it's a story about people.' She says the book that got her into love stories was *The Flatshare* by Beth O'Leary. 'It was as simple as *loving* these characters so much and wanting them to be together. The premise – Tilly and Leon getting to know each other as they share a bed, before they've *actually* met, is clever. But it's Tilly and Leon themselves that make the story great.'

Becki has theories about why readers in their teens and 20s are embracing romance. 'We read because it's hard to find the romance we crave in real life. I think it's getting really hard to meet anyone in real life and spend time with them,' she says. 'I live with my parents and I'd love to move out, but that's not going to be possible for a while. My big sister is still at home and she hasn't dated much. She started uni in 2020 – she was really excited about living away from home and having some kind of love life, but obviously the pandemic made that difficult. I think it's affected me too.' She adds 'I hate to say it, but a lot of the people I'm attracted to in real life are quite disappointing. In books, everyone is hotter and smarter!'

In my teens, my parents would have *loved* it if I'd chosen books over dates, but there has been much analysis, and anxiety, over Gen Z dating trends. A survey from dating app Hinge found that 90 per cent of Gen Z users fear rejection, and 25 per cent are less confident on a first date since the pandemic.[8] Gen Z has been credited with making the sales of romance novels soar,[9] but do they prefer dates on the page to love in real life? And should we be worried?

Sex and relationships expert Nichi Hodgson writes that maybe we're all just getting fussier – and that's a good thing. 'Consent, connection, mutual respect, a narrowing of the orgasm gap, are more than buzzwords: they are the standards by which we now measure the best intimate encounters.'[10] Perhaps the younger romance readers are using fantasy to shape their expectations of reality. When we read romance novels, we learn how we'd like to be treated and how we'd like to feel when we're with a partner.

Readers like Becki *should* have high standards for real-life love. In the 21st century, women aren't waiting for men to propose marriage and guarantee their economic safety, yet equally old-fashioned heteronormative values still linger. If love stories make women fussy about who they choose to be with, instead of waiting to be chosen, then the romance trend could have life-changing benefits.

Worried in love

For a long time, my romantic life was filled with anxiety. As a lonely, self-conscious teenager, I could be heard complaining, 'It was all right for Juliet, at least she *had* a boyfriend.' I was desperate for romance, but I didn't have any confidence in my ability to attract it. Falling in love and having someone fall in love with me was my greatest dream – and I was convinced that there was no way it could come true. I was full of feelings and while reading about love strengthened those feelings, it also eased them and made them slightly more manageable.

In *The Pursuit of Love* by Nancy Mitford, Linda decides that she's in love with the Prince of Wales, and Fanny, the narrator, then falls 'in love' with a farmer she's seen out in the fields, from a distance. Neither character has ever met the person they're 'in love' with, but they *might*, and they're so overwhelmed with a sense of passion that they both need to be 'in love' with *someone*. 'These loves were strong, and painfully delicious; they occupied all our thoughts. They were to keep the house warm, so to speak, for its eventual occupant.'[11] Mitford's observation brought me much comfort. I might be alone, but I wasn't alone in my yearning, even if that yearning had no specific object.

But perhaps the greatest impact that *The Pursuit of Love* had on me was its exploration of love in and out of marriage. It's a romantic comedy about women falling for men, but it does not pitch marriage as an end in itself. Linda's relationship with Tony Kroesig, which ends in divorce, would now be called a 'starter marriage', but in 1935, when the novel was published, the divorce rate was extremely low.[12] The Matrimonial Clause Act, which allowed women to petition for divorce on the same grounds as men, wasn't made law until 1937. Linda gets married for a second time, and this also ends in disaster. When she finally meets the love of her life, Fabrice, she does not marry him.

It still seems radical to me that this happens to a woman in an 80-year-old book. Linda's upper-class privileges grant her a lot of freedom, but she's allowed her flaws. She makes mistakes. She can't have her coup de foudre until she's known what it's like to fall out of love. Like Juliet, Linda dies for love, in a way (spoiler alert), while giving birth to Fabrice's baby.

Other characters feared that Linda's future was foreshadowed by her aunt, 'the Bolter' – nicknamed for her tendency to bolt away from one marriage straight into another. 'Bolting' is an act that does not go unpunished. The women in the story are teased and shamed in turns, but there's a delicious sense of defiance in Linda's character. She isn't a traditional 'good girl', but she gets to be the heroine. She thinks of herself first, she lives for love, and she isn't willing to sacrifice her sense of self by sticking around and trying to make the best of a bad marriage. *The Pursuit of Love* stands out for me because it's one of the few classic novels in which love doesn't lead women to sadness and sacrifice. For Linda, true love feels like freedom.

I still pick up *The Pursuit of Love* when I'm feeling anxious, although now, I'm just as drawn to the other love story that rumbles along quietly in the background. Cousin Fanny, the narrator, finds lasting love with Alfred, an undemonstrative Oxford don.[13] We're not shown much of Fanny's life with Alfred, but we can guess what it's like. It seems steady, and secure. She doesn't have much to report. When we meet her, she's a wise child who feels like an outsider. She's not quite as dashing or glamorous as her wild cousins, but as she matures and marries Alfred, her voice changes. She's still Fanny, but she seems to grow in quiet confidence. She becomes clear-eyed. She narrates Linda's escapades with love and interest, but she's not standing in Linda's shadow in the same way.

This is very lifelike. When our own relationships are unhappily dramatic, there is much to discuss. Before I met Dale, I was briefly, miserably, and one-sidedly in love with someone who made it very clear that he was not interested in me. He was never my boyfriend – at the time, it didn't even feel right to say I was 'seeing' him *because I barely saw him*. Yet, this man warranted hours of analysis! I talked about him to everyone all the time. To me, it felt like a storybook love affair because the highs were dizzying and the lows were crushing. I was capable of creating enough drama for two all by myself.

When I met Dale, I learned that love stories don't need to be dramatic or tragic. I stopped telling my story because I was too happy and too busy living it. And I was learning a very important lesson. My anxiety and unhappiness weren't curses. I wasn't doomed to one sort of relationship (bad) with one sort of person (bad) because there was something wrong with me. However, I tended to behave like the heroine of a bad book. I'd been waiting to be chosen and rescued. If someone else found me desirable, likeable, and lovable, I could become those things. I thought my value depended on the endorsement of a difficult man – a Darcy, a Heathcliff, a person whose affection was worthy because it was hard to win.

'Happily ever after'

The stories we read, and the stories we're told, tend to elevate romantic love as being the best and most significant kind of love. It is presented as the main event in any human life. We share stories about looking for love and when we've found it, the story ends.

We don't venerate the other kinds of love in the same way or put them on a pedestal. There are love stories about families and friendships. There are stories about how we struggle to learn to love ourselves. These stories don't get the same size audience as *Romeo and Juliet*, but I think they're just as interesting, just as captivating. I'm a romantic and I want to believe that love is the answer and conquers all. I'm also a human who believes love is deeper, richer, and much more complex than that. I want to know how love evolves and how we evolve with it. I want to read stories about how romantic love shouldn't become your whole life, but can make other love even stronger and brighter. I want to know what happens after we fall in love.

My love story started when I realised I wasn't simply the love interest, I was interesting all by myself. I wasn't just a girlfriend, I'd found someone who treated me as an equal partner, a co-star, a fellow adventurer. I'll always adore reading romances, but sometimes they tell us that love is agony, anxiety, and uncertainty. A woman in love can't eat or sleep. In the stories we read, people *die* for love.

But in my real-life story, I live for it.

'The most satisfying moments are the moments of yearning, before anything actually happens'

If anyone knows anything about love stories, it's bestselling novelist and screenwriter David Nicholls. David is best known for the global smash hit *One Day*, the story of Emma and Dexter. I've been captivated by every single one of David's novels. He's also adapted several novels for screen, including Thomas Hardy's *Far from the Madding Crowd.* David and I talked about writing about love, reading about love, and why we're so captivated by romance on the page.

I want to know how it feels to write a love story that readers respond to so strongly. *One Day* is part of the contemporary canon; it's a novel that we keep reading, watching, and wondering about. David explains that *One Day* is never far away. 'At the moment, I'm touring with my new book, *You Are Here*, but when we get to the Q&A part of the event, everyone wants to ask me about the ending of *One Day*. This didn't happen when the novel was first published. Everyone accepted the ending then; no one said, "Did you mean to do this?" or even "How dare you do this!"'

David has a theory. 'I think this is because of the recent Netflix adaptation. I think people feel so connected to the actors [Ambika Mod and Leo Woodall] and they're much, much more upset when the "happy ending" is snatched away.' David has mixed feelings about this. I suggest it shows how powerful his work is and how intensely people are responding to the characters he has created. 'I must admit, I'm finding it quite hard, because I never thought of changing that ending. And if it didn't have that ending, I don't think we'd both be talking about the book right now.'

David and I wrack our brains, trying to find examples of love stories in literature that end happily. 'Maybe happy endings are especially difficult on the page because it's hard to get the kind of rush and satisfaction that you feel when they're on screen,' he suggests. 'Perhaps the one I know best is in *Far from the Madding Crowd* – it's a happy ending that is occurring in the future. It's about the potential for happiness.'

When we speak, David is helping his children with revision for their exams and tells me that he's returned to the work of the queen of the romcom, Jane Austen. 'I don't always get on with Austen because I struggle with the inevitability of the stories. There aren't really any surprises in the arc of *Pride and Prejudice*.

But then we know the story before we've read the story. We can't come to it anew. It's one of the original "enemies to lovers" premises, I suppose.'

I ask David about his novel *Us*, a book I love. It's a story about the end of a 25-year relationship, the couple taking one last holiday – a grand tour of Europe – with their teenage son. I suggest that I don't think it's about a 'failed' marriage, but one that comes to an end when it's supposed to. 'I wanted to write about the end of a marriage in a way that wasn't acrimonious,' he explains. 'Divorce, especially in fiction, is always bitter, angry, and to do with infidelity. This was my attempt to see if it could happen tenderly. Of course, it's a comedy, so things have to get heightened and pained, but the actual decision feels humane, I think.'

David is interested in the writers who explore relationships beyond the 'happily ever after'. 'Katherine Heiny writes about love and relationships in a way that's really fond and strong. Maybe I'd like to write another marriage novel and try to capture that flirtiness and lightness. I don't like it when novels are overly poetic about love, or when they talk about it as though it's some kind of spell or when there's a fatalistic inevitability about it.'

Perhaps this comes back to the trouble with Austen – that we readers know, before we pick the book up, the couple is going to get together, no matter how unlikely it seems, and so we lose the sense of surprise. And we lose our connection with the characters. We want to be discovering their love and falling with them. We don't want to feel that we know more than they do or they know more than us. 'I've never got on with magic realism or anything overly spiritual about love because I've wanted to know what the characters are laughing about together. Are they teasing each other about anything? You want to see the connection grow over time. It's no fun if they look at each other and instantly think "Well, that's it." *Especially* when it's because they see physical perfection in each other, and it suggests love is something they have no say in or control over. I think real attraction is very different from that.'

I agree with David and, as readers, we both feel that it's hard to get this on the page. 'I'm often asked to talk about the "great" love stories and I have to say that I find it really difficult to think of any because so many of them are so frustrating. The characters are rarely together on the page. You look at *The Great Gatsby* or *Doctor Zhivago* and it's all about separation, obstacles, and yearning, but never really a sense of love building. Or watching the experience of love. Reading about it can be a bit like watching people kiss in the park. You think "good for you", but it's not really for me. And in all literature, once anyone actually gets together, it all goes to hell. The most satisfying moments are the moments of yearning, before anything actually happens.'

Does our idea of ideal romantic love change over time, I wonder? And does our definition of romance change? 'A lot of the love stories I used to respond to as a younger man were pretty poisonous,' David tells me. '*Tender Is the Night* by F. Scott Fitzgerald is about an abusive relationship, a doctor who takes advantage of a vulnerable patient. There are moments of great lyricism and beauty and, superficially, it's a portrait of a glamorous, exciting couple. *Tess of the D'Urbervilles* is a book that obsessed me as a teenager. But Hardy's novels are full of those awful moments where you think, "Oh no, this is a *really* bad idea. And there's *Great Expectations*. I loved it, and I still love it, but there's nothing tender or loving in it.'

David is curious about the way the American 20th-century novelists have shaped our understanding of romance and relationships. 'Those stories about love, sex, and relationships tend to be so focused on infidelity and adultery. *Light Years* by James Salter is a very good novel about love in a marriage and the reality of marriage. But it's also about anxiety, ageing, and fear of the future. It's very real.'

David's most recent novel, *You Are Here*, explores these themes too. It's the story of Marnie and Michael, who are unusual protagonists for a love story in that they're respectively in their late 30s and early 40s. They come to us, the readers, with disappointments, grief, life experience – and some reluctance to look for love at all. 'When we use the phrase "love story", we think of something with high stakes, like *Romeo and Juliet* or *Titanic*, and *You Are Here* might be the story of two people trying to work out whether they're on a date.' I tell him that I love the authenticity of that. Perhaps there's a place for drama and escapism, and we can lose ourselves in idealised portrayals of love, but we also crave the quietly profound and we need to read love stories that reflect the truth of human experience.

Like me, David loves reading the novels of Marian Keyes and suggests her most recent book, *My Favourite Mistake*, is a good example of this. 'It feels very hopeful to have a story about mature people finding themselves and connecting with each other.'

How reading brings love into my life

Reading about relationships can help us to understand more about who we are and who we're drawn to. Do you love Mr Darcy because he's distant and remote or because he's ultimately principled and kind – or because you wish you were Lizzie Bennett? This is something to think about before you fall for the next person who ignores you at a party.

Love stories help me to view the world through a more romantic lens and make me notice and appreciate expressions of love in my life. I don't expect anyone to slay a dragon for me, but I'm thrilled when they make me a cup of tea.

Love stories *should* raise our standards. When we read, it's easy to notice when someone is being treated with a lack of respect and kindness – the story might be fictional, but our values are real. We deserve to be treated just as well as our favourite characters.

My favourite books about love

Early Morning Riser by Katherine Heiny

When Jane moves to Michigan, she instantly falls for Duncan – handsome, good-natured, and charming. In fact, every other woman in Boyne City seems to have succumbed to Duncan's charms at one point or another. This is an incredibly funny, generous, huge-hearted book about what happens when you find a way to love people for exactly who they are. It's a story about when romantic love finds its biggest, deepest expression and encompasses everyone your partner cares about too.

Larry's Party by Carol Shields

We meet Larry when he's 26, and this novel follows him all the way into his 50s, through three romantic relationships. It's written with exquisite depth and lightness. It's a very simple, real story about emotional life and the way our feelings can fade and swell over time. It's remarkable for its ordinariness, a quietly beautiful book about romance, mistakes, and the hope that sustains us all in our quest for lasting love.

Us by David Nicholls

Connie and Douglas have been married for 25 years when Connie tells Douglas that, as their son, Albie, is ready to leave home for college, she thinks their marriage might have run its course. A devastated Douglas decides that their last family holiday together, a grand tour of Europe, might give Connie a reason to fall in love with him all over again. This beautiful, wise book examines the mechanics of a marriage intimately. It's a subtle, thoughtful exploration of how love waxes and wanes, and what happens beyond 'happily ever after'.

Wedding Toasts I'll Never Give by Ada Calhoun

This is a smart, funny, tender essay collection about romantic hyperbole and the realities of making a life and building a family with someone when you both have passions, dreams, careers, and relationship histories. It's pragmatic but joyous, real but hopeful. 'There is so much beauty in the trying, and in the failing, and in the trying again,' she writes. 'Epic failure is part of being human, and it's definitely part of being married.'[14] Amen.

Everything I Know About Love by **Dolly Alderton**

Alderton's smash hit memoir is a romcom with a twist – a book about one woman's fascination with romantic love and how, in the course of her search for romance, she finds there's already deep, meaningful love in her life – in her relationships with her friends, family, and even herself. It's funny, moving, and beautiful, and should be prescribed reading for anyone who has ever loved anyone or anything. I often think that if only someone had given this book to Juliet, Shakespeare would have been forced to write a very different ending.

9
Reading like a
WRITER

"Read, read, read. Read everything – trash, classics, good and bad, and see how they do it... Then write"

William Faulkner[1]

I'm standing in the shower, listening to Adam Buxton's podcast as I wash my hair. He makes a reference to 'Vinyl justice', a segment on his TV programme, *The Adam and Joe Show*, in which he and Joe Cornish would turn up at pop stars' houses, dressed as police officers, and demand to go through their record collections. I think about what would happen if someone turned up now, to inspect the cultural contents of my flat. The first thing they would see were the books. The bookcase in the hall and the pile of books beside it, which is currently taller than I am. The books in the bedroom, the books in the kitchen. The spare room, with three big bookcases, and piles of books on the desk. The books next to the toilet.

What would this mysterious inspector make of this lack of order? Tolstoy beside Denis Johnson beside *The Jolly Postman*. Every book is a record of a whim, a moment of curiosity, and connection. A splurge in Waterstones, a discovery in a charity shop, or a gift – a token of someone else's love and thoughtfulness.

I'm a writer. Dale is a writer. That's why we have so many books. It dawns on me that we're writers *because* we're readers. Our collection is unique. Every other writer will probably have an unusual, eclectic collection of books too. Every other writer is inspired by a combination of other writers. And yet, their voices are as unique as their bookshelves. The writers I love and learn from are the ones who have distinct voices. I wonder about the writers that inspired them and helped them to find those voices.

What if I was a book inspector? If I went to writers' houses and looked at *their* shelves, what would I find? I bet I'd discover some of my favourite books, and some of my future favourite books. I think it would be fascinating.

I bet at least *one* Booker Prize winner also has a copy of *The Jolly Postman*.

The idea makes me tingle. I'm not going to let this lie. I think there are some exciting conversations to come about the connection between reading stories and telling them. I dream, and then I plan. Over the coming months, these conversations start to happen and we record them. A year later, the first episode of You're Booked, with Dolly Alderton, is launched.

Your secret storytelling powers

All readers are writers. If you're reading this book, you're a writer. If you're a human with a phone in the 21st century, you're a writer. If you've ever written an Instagram caption, you're a writer. If your personal or professional life involves communicating with anyone, in any way, *you're a writer*. It doesn't matter how you did in your exams, what your teachers told you, or if you have the first 10,000 words of a novel hidden on an old laptop, and you've been trying not to think about it for the last five years, *you're a writer*. You have a voice.

And that makes you a storyteller.

Why do I want you to know this?

Because so many of us find that all our interactions are fraught with anxiety – from working on a creative project, to giving a presentation, to sending a difficult email. And when we find ways to feel confident about how we communicate, we're able to cage and manage that anxiety. There have never been more demands on our attention, and that can make it hard to seek attention when we need to. Sometimes we all worry that we're not interesting, we're not worthy, and we don't have anything to say. But when you feel confident about your storytelling powers, you'll know that you are interesting. You'll realise you have something to say that's worth listening to. And your audience – whether that's one person or 10,000 people – will believe you and believe in you. Tapping into that confidence can free you from the pressure to get your message 'right', so you can concentrate on finding your unique voice and discovering what it is that makes you sound like you.

Reading widely teaches us that stories don't necessarily need to be dramatic to be fascinating. If a storyteller has a compelling voice, we pay attention. When we read, we learn how stories are told, and how sometimes it's the telling itself that makes us pay attention. The best books remind us that this power lies within us.

How stories shape us

I work with a wide range of writers and readers. I teach a fiction-writing course, and I mentor authors, guiding them as they develop their ideas and find their voices. I also work with people who don't necessarily want to write a book right now but want to become more confident as communicators. And I've got good news for them, and you: every story you've ever engaged with has enriched your skills and abilities. Most of us have been studying the art of storytelling all our lives. You already have a unique set of references and influences – everything you need to help you discover your voice.

When we spend time with children, we share stories with them. We might read to them – and they might come to us with requests. They might engage our transcription services, or employ us as actors. I've 'made' books with my nieces and nephews – they've told me what they want the story to be, I've written it down, and stapled it together. I've improvised a story about pirates and one robot-pirate, a storm, and an enchanted treasure chest. Children generate ideas relentlessly. They improvise. They're not worried about endings, pacing, or whether everything has been done before. They don't worry about whether their story is worthy of our attention because we're adults – it's our job to pay attention to them! They're so absorbed by the worlds they have created that there's simply no room for doubt. Most importantly, almost every book they read makes them want to create a story of their own. It never occurs to them that storytelling requires status or that they need to work and wait to start speaking. Enthusiasm and ideas are the only qualifications they need.

Instinctive storytelling

We might not remember the first story we told, but maybe we can recall the breathless urgency of that moment. The feeling that the story was a storm, shaking us, and sharing it was the only way to restore ourselves to calm. Or perhaps we can remember feeling playful – the wonder of not knowing how our stories were going to end and the sense that we were going to have fun finding out. These feelings are probably worlds away from the heavy dread you feel when you think about clicking through your slides on Microsoft Teams next Tuesday afternoon. But you can recapture the magic of being excited to tell a story as soon as you start to understand the way that you've been forged by stories.

As we get older, we start to worry about all the ways that we can get things wrong. We stop looking for opportunities to tell stories because of our fear of failure. We feel judged, vulnerable, and exposed, and we start to second-guess ourselves. We get in our own way because we know that we'll never be able to express our ideas perfectly, and we'll never meet our own high standards, so we stop trying. It took me a long time to learn that I had to step into my anxiety and sit with my fear if I was ever going to release the stories that were building up inside me. And I'm still learning that the only way to get good at storytelling is to practise.

Anyone can write

When I wrote my first novel, I was overwhelmed by anxiety. I worried that I wasn't a good enough writer. I was convinced that there was a secret science involved in storytelling and I could never master it. Characters and situations kept inviting themselves into my brain and I didn't know what to do with them. What if I couldn't do them justice? The action wouldn't be dramatic enough, the ending wouldn't be satisfying enough. I could come up with a beginning, then a thick fog would descend. I didn't know what I was doing, I didn't know anything about acts, scenes, timing. I can't read maps or understand the instructions that come with flat-pack furniture. There was no way I could build an imaginary world.

So how did I overcome my fears? And why do I want you to know that you can write a novel, if you want to?

I reached a tipping point. My fear of not writing became greater than the fear of trying. I realised that I had to risk failure because the alternative was worse. It meant stepping around my greatest dream, trying to ignore it, gritting my teeth as the itch became itchier the more I refused to scratch. The urge, the wish, took up space in my brain, swelling up and squeezing out everything else. I worried that everything had been done before and I'd never be able to write anything original. Then I thought about the books I loved, and the way they overlapped, echoing one another, borrowing from one another. Yes, everything had been done before. But it hadn't been done by me. I had a voice too. It was time to use it.

Learning from books

When I was stuck on my first draft, I interviewed the multi-million-selling novelist Julie Cohen for the You're Booked podcast. Julie told me two things that stuck in my head. First, she'd written some novels for Mills & Boon (and her very first novel for them was rejected). Second, she believed she'd learned the most about writing novels when she was a teacher and taught the same books on rotation for a whole term at a time. 'You know more than you think,' she said, when I told her my woes. 'If you read a lot of novels, you absorb everything you need to know about plot and pacing. And when you go back to the same story repeatedly, you learn a lot. There's always something new to spot.'[2]

I left Julie's bookshelves with a spring in my step. My shoulders had dropped from up by my ears. I didn't need to worry that I wasn't good enough, I wasn't prepared enough, and that I didn't know enough. I'd been getting ready to write a novel since I was three years old. Every time I woke up in the middle of the night and read myself back to sleep with a familiar story, I was learning. I didn't need to take a year off to do an MA, read a lot of technical books, or even wait until I had a doctor's note that proclaimed my anxiety had been cured for ever. All I had to do was sit with the story that had entered my head and see what happened. I knew what made a story captivating because I'd spent so much of my life feeling captivated by stories.

Julie had answered a question I'd been subconsciously asking for months. I loved talking about books. Deep down, I hoped that if I spent enough time rubbing shoulders with novelists, I could 'catch' fiction. Someone would take pity on me and share the secret. 'I used to experience soul-crushing anxiety too!' they'd say. 'The idea of writing gave me panic attacks! But then, I tried eating a whole head of lettuce a day/praying to Lupus, the pagan wolf god/getting good and drunk, and I was fine! Apparently, Saul Bellow did it!'

Curious writers

As I interviewed more writers, I started to understand the way that they read. They had open minds, and hearts. They had a thirst for novelty, an unquenchable curiosity, and a sentimental streak. Dolly Alderton was forever altered by the illustrations in *The Joy of Sex*, having sneaked glimpses of her mother's copy when she had moments alone in the house. Stuart Heritage kept a copy of *Cookin' with Coolio*, simply because it existed and it brought him joy every time he saw it on the shelf. Cathy Rentzenbrink still had the paperback copy of *Pride and Prejudice* that she first read when she was 15. Jess Phillips showed me her treasured copy of *The Secret Diary of Adrian Mole Aged 13¾* and told me that she wished Pauline Mole could run the country. Elif Shafak showed us her rolling library ladder, like Belle's in *Beauty and the Beast*, and told of her passion for *Don Quixote*. Marian Keyes reads romance when the world feels a little too much for her, and believes that reading exactly what you want to read, when you want to read it, is medicinal.

Also, if we want to tell a particular kind of story, it makes sense to read that kind of story. Study a thriller and you'll soon discover what makes it thrilling. Every writer I spoke to was omnivorous. The more widely they read, the more curious they became, and they used that curiosity as fuel for their own work. Reading was a source of pleasure, comfort, and relaxation, but they couldn't help learning something about their craft when they did it, even if they were simply reading a book to their children.

Most importantly, every writer I spoke to told me that reading is a vital part of their writing practice. They didn't read every day, and they didn't love everything that they read. Some had been reading voraciously for as long as they could remember. Some had fallen out of love with reading and found their way back to books. Together, they taught me that there was no right way to read but, as long as they were reading, they were stoking the fire that made them want to tell and share stories.

Confident communicating

Storytelling is an ancient practice. We still use motifs from ancient myths and fables to illustrate, explain, and understand our lives. Every time I write, I try to channel the tortoise. I know there's a word count and a deadline in sight, and the only way to get to the finish line is by plodding slowly and consistently, not thinking about the hypothetical hare, who can write much faster than me. 'Slow and steady wins the race' is something I must tell myself most days. This means that I'm regularly taking writing advice that is more than 2,000 years old. 'The Hare and the Tortoise' is believed to be one of Aesop's famous fables. Aesop was a slave who lived in ancient Greece, around 600BC.[3] His stories were told rather than written and were passed down the generations.

We read to sate our craving for stories. We're also continually learning how to become better storytellers. You might want to learn how to write a novel. You also might want to learn how to capture everyone's attention in a meeting, what to say when you bump into your neighbour, or how to feel more confident when you post on social media. Every time you read, you're developing those resources. You're increasing your vocabulary and finding out how to become a more confident communicator. You're learning about how you respond to language and discovering new ways to use it.

Finding your voice

Berta, 35, says, 'About a year ago, I was promoted, and my new role involved giving a *lot* of presentations. This made me so anxious. I don't think I'd ever experienced imposter syndrome before. I'd faced plenty of challenges at work, but I'd always been able to overcome them with research and preparation. The idea of speaking in front of people was terrifying. What if I didn't have enough information? What if I got it wrong or people felt bored? I started making these very dense, fact-packed presentations, and I could tell that everyone was as miserable watching them as I was when I was giving them.'

Berta explains that her mother helped her to realise that she had strong storytelling skills, she just needed to rediscover them. 'I was talking to my mum about how anxious I was becoming, and that the situation seemed to be getting worse, not better. She said, "It's so funny because, when you were little, you loved presentations." She reminded me that I'd really enjoyed giving book reports at school and that I'd often give them at home, just for fun. I was perfectly happy when I was talking about a story and I felt confident about sharing information – it never occurred to me that it was something you could be good or bad at, I just did it.'

Berta decided to challenge herself and try to find a story within the information she had to share. 'I realised that I couldn't go on unless I discovered a way to make the presentations a little bit more engaging. And that the way to bring the information to life was to find some points of human connection and give the presentation some shape. Instead of simply sharing as much data as I could, I had to find a creative way to interpret it. I still get slightly anxious, and there are limits when it comes to making a presentation entertaining. No deck about marketing techniques is ever going to be as captivating as *Fantastic Mr Fox*, but I've learned that the way I tell the story of the content is just as important as the content itself. In fact, I've always known that. I just needed to be reminded of it.'

Perfectionism and fear

Jerry Seinfeld tells a joke about public speaking being the average person's number one fear – with number two being death – so suggests that most of us would rather be inside the coffin than standing beside it delivering the eulogy. Many of us, though, will find ourselves in a situation like Berta's, where we'll have to stand up and speak, even though it makes us feel deeply anxious. Perfectionism rears its head. We imagine all the ways we can get it wrong, the negative things people will say, and how quickly we'll fail. But we *can* cope with the experience, and even enjoy it, if we learn to trust our storytelling skills. When I need to give a presentation, I feel the pressure to make it flawless, but stories aren't flawless. Reading reminds me there's no such thing as a perfect story or a perfect storyteller. All we need to do is keep our audience curious.

Equally, our written communication can cause anxiety. An Australian study found that the average office worker sends 40 emails a day.[4] We're all writing, all the time, but that doesn't mean we find it easy. We're overwhelmed by the volume of information we receive and share.[5] We find different voices and become different versions of ourselves. On any given day, we might be emailing managers, landlords, and our partners. I've spent an hour staring at the words 'Dear X, I hope you're really well' because I'm not sure which tone to use for an email to an editor over an unpaid invoice. It can be very hard to inject the right amount of warmth and humanity into an email in these situations and be appropriately respectful. I'm not sure any of us get it right consistently. So when I receive an email that seems a little chilly, I cheer myself up by remembering that it's no reflection on me, and probably not on the sender – it's just the nature of emails.

Reading about writing

There are many excellent, practical books about writing, storytelling, and creating work for an audience. Many You're Booked guests have told me that it's been helpful for them to read *about* writing, even though they largely feel that the best way to learn how to tell stories is to read stories themselves.

The book I recommend to everyone starting a writing project is *Big Magic* by Elizabeth Gilbert. This changed the way I felt about writing – and reading. Gilbert is an advocate of finding pure pleasure in our creative practice, and this book taught me to look for joy and to trust in it.

Gilbert writes, 'The Greeks and Romans both believed in an external daemon of creativity... the Romans called it your genius. The Romans didn't believe an exceptionally gifted person was a genius, they believed an exceptionally gifted person *had* a genius.'[6] Gilbert theorises that our geniuses come and go, and we can't rely on their presence or take them for granted. We simply have to notice when they appear and make the most of our time with them – trying to keep working even when they are nowhere to be seen. My genius seems to be a long way from my desk today, but I know that if I simply sit still and keep storytelling, it will come back. I certainly don't want it to accuse me of slacking off. And I believe that every time I lose myself in a different story, my genius becomes curious. It finds a new reason to show up to work.

Big Magic is a story about storytelling. How it's done and *why* it's done. Every time I read it, I find something new and inspiring within it, but it reminds me of the same simple truth every time: any story is worth telling as long as we want to tell it. We don't need to prove ourselves or prove the value of our stories. But every time we share a story, we become stronger.

Another book to boost your confidence and reignite the joy of storytelling is *Bird by Bird* by Anne Lamott. The title comes from the writing advice given by Lamott's father to her big brother, who was writing through tears, struggling to finish a school project about birds that he'd had three months to write. 'Bird by bird, buddy. Just take it bird by bird.'[7]

What does this mean? It's advice that captures the sense of precisely why storytelling is so daunting. Before we begin, we're panicking about whether we'll ever be able to get to the end. We're impatient – I believe impatience is a form of fear. Have you ever rushed your speech because you're worried that the person you're talking to is getting bored and annoyed? Have you ever had an idea that presented itself to you like an unlit firework, then instantly dismissed it because you were worried that you wouldn't have enough time or resources to light it up and project it into the air? Have you ever tried to meditate while your brain is saying, 'Is it over yet? Is it over yet? Is it over yet? How can 10 minutes be *so long?*'

I suspect it's never been harder to be present, but it's never been more important to try. If we can take all our stories 'bird by bird', we free ourselves from the future perfect. We release ourselves from the anxiety that we might be wasting someone's time. Describing your bird will take as long as it takes. You don't need to worry about how to get to the next bird, you just need to trust that it's there. It will be ready for you when the time is right.

Lamott is keen to demystify the process of writing and storytelling. 'It's a matter of persistence and faith and hard work. So you might as well just go ahead and get started.'[8] Yes, storytelling is a latent talent – we can all do it and do it well. But it's also a skill, and the only way to build a skill is to keep practising it. This is why reading is such a powerful part of the work. I can always learn something from the way someone else tells a story.

Another book that had a huge impact on my confidence and storytelling skills was *Four Thousand Weeks* by Oliver Burkeman. The title comes from the average human lifespan – that is, if we're lucky, we each get about 4,000 weeks on Earth. Burkeman's book is about his struggle to do more in less time, but it's also a meditative, generous, and compelling exploration of our obsession with creativity, completion, deadlines, and endings. Burkeman speaks to all of us when he writes, 'even those of us who were bookworms as children now struggle to make it through a paragraph without reaching for our phones'.[9]

If storytelling feels difficult, and you're struggling to sustain the attention of your audience, it's probably not your fault. It's because it's incredibly hard for us to reach one another when our attention is so fractured. The people we speak to don't reach for their phones because they're bored but because they're scared. What if something has gone wrong elsewhere in their lives? What if they miss an urgent, angry message from their boss or perhaps there's a childcare issue they're concerned about, or they don't know how to get home.

Burkeman's book is enormously reassuring, as it suggests theories explaining why we're all struggling to focus and might struggle to get anyone to focus on us. It doesn't matter how brilliant your story is, or how well you're telling it, you have absolutely no control over the state of mind of the listener. Chances are, they're going to be distracted. So you can release yourself from the pressure to tell the best story ever. You can also practise paying attention to stories and become an invaluable, generous listener.

It's easy to argue that reading can soothe our anxiety. When I suggest that you find comfort in books when you're feeling nervous, frazzled, or frightened, I'm telling you to take it easy.

It's a suggestion to spend some time alone, enjoying the quiet, escaping your fear, and having permission to amble around someone else's universe. Reading alone is relaxing. We know this.

But, for many of us, the idea that reading could be a gateway drug to writing, holding our own at parties, and even public speaking will bring the anxiety running back to torment us. How could I suggest such a thing?

In theory, we can deal with anxiety indefinitely if we avoid any situation that might trigger it. However, in the long run, this approach isn't sustainable. When we're scared of experiencing anxiety or stress, we don't develop the skills we need to deal with those feelings. Also, when we're stressed, our bodies release adrenaline and cortisol, sometimes causing us to experience physical symptoms. Anxiety comes with raised temperatures and upset stomachs, so if you feel nervous about a party, you might end up not feeling well enough to go anyway.

But this approach has other effects too. When we avoid anything that might make us anxious, we start to shrink our world. We stop growing, challenging ourselves, and looking for adventure. This is why stories are vital. They make us look upwards and outside ourselves. We learn about people living with fear and moving beyond it. And when we tell our stories, we align ourselves with those people and discover strength in numbers. When we put ourselves in some of the situations that scare us, and survive, we learn that we're so much more powerful than our anxiety. We begin to build a confidence that no one can take away from us.

When you read, you're never stuck for something to do or something to say. You don't have to tell your own story – you can share elements of the stories that you've engaged with and responded to. Elizabeth Gilbert's story about having a genius in *Big Magic* is borrowed from the ancient Romans. Anne Lamott's career-defining bird story is borrowed from her father and brother.

If you can get back in touch with the part of yourself that breathed stories, you can start to change your life. You'll learn that your anxiety is survivable. You'll be able to get past the sharp fear you feel at the start of a work presentation. You'll be able to walk into any room, in any building, alone, and know that you can speak to anyone you meet. You'll also light up the lives of your friends and family by becoming a better speaker and listener.

There was a time when my anxiety felt like a prison. I struggled to find the strength to fight it. I was always trying to hide from it, yet it always managed to find me. It estranged me from myself. It made me believe that I couldn't be touched by hope or joy. I let myself listen to the story it wanted to tell me. It told me to try to become smaller. It told me not to try.

But when life felt dark, sad, and small, I still had stories. I knew this couldn't be my ending; I knew I couldn't stay this way for ever. I was being held captive by the White Queen. In anxiety land, it was always winter, but never Christmas. I found ways to melt the snow. I realised that I could bear anything for a minute, then an hour at a time, and I suspected that something wonderful might be waiting for me on the other side of the anxiety barrier. The only way to change the story was to take charge of the story. I had to make something happen. The anxiety wasn't going to leave unless I showed it that I wanted it to go.

We worry about whether we have any right to tell our imperfect stories. How can we begin if we don't know what the ending will be? But that's precisely why we all need to become storytellers: we can't find out unless we start.

Summoning your inner storyteller – how writing and reading can build your creative confidence

- **Find out what your favourite writers read** The authors you love are inspired by the authors they love, so go to the source and expose yourself to their influences. Most authors share their favourite books on social media and talk about the writers they love in interviews. If you're not sure where to begin, the You're Booked podcast archives are a great place to start!

• **Think about all the ways you communicate** Who makes you laugh in your group chat? Whose emails do you look forward to? Who is the clearest, most direct person you know? These people are using storytelling methods to get their messages across. Think about why their words have impact and are effective.

• **Be clear and sincere** Don't worry about being clever or entertaining; just make sure that you're being straightforward and the people you're addressing can understand and follow you. Trust that your flair and personality will rise to the surface and shine over time. Once you feel confident in the basics, you'll begin to find opportunities to be creative and playful.

• **Practice makes perfect** When it comes to telling stories, we can't build on our skills unless we're willing to speak up and put ourselves forward. We learn by doing, sharing, and trying. If we can step into our fear and have a go even if we're worried that we're not very good, we'll eventually become great.

Books to help you find your voice

On Writing by Stephen King

King's book, 'part memoir, part masterclass' is frequently cited by authors as a major source of inspiration. It's great on how to master the art of storytelling with confidence and clarity. It's also excellent on maintaining your equilibrium and sense of self in the face of adversity. This is one of the most commonly mentioned books on the You're Booked podcast. Holly Bourne, Dorothy Koomson, Jessica Knoll, Steve Jones, D. B. C. Pierre, and Janina Matthewson are all fans.

Mortification by Robin Robertson

This painfully funny book is a collection of anecdotes from iconic authors – ranging from Margaret Atwood to Julian Barnes – recalling their worst moments of public shame in their professional life. This is a book about storytelling, vulnerability, and having a sense of humour about yourself. All vital qualities for developing your own distinctive voice.

Your Story Matters by Nikesh Shukla

This beautiful, generous, encouraging book will guide you towards discovering your voice and help you to sound like yourself when you write – whether you have plans for a novel, an essay, or just a very important Post-it note. It's great for boosting your confidence – it will make you feel as though there's someone in your corner cheering you on.

10

Reading beyond your comfort zone
(and returning to it)

"It is very difficult to be learned; it seems as if people were worn out on the way to great thoughts and can never enjoy them because they are too tired"

George Eliot[1]

I've been reading the same page for about half an hour. I shift on my sunlounger. I sigh, I squint. I smudge the book with sunscreen. Come on, Daisy. This is Norman Mailer. He's a very important writer. *The Naked and the Dead* is a classic. It's part of the contemporary canon.

I try again. I'm distracted by a mosquito. I can do this. I'll get to the end of the chapter, then I'll have an ice cream. Focus! Focus on the Second World War. I start the page again. But then I think, '*Hold on. I'm on holiday!*' One day, I'll be ready for *The Naked and the Dead*, but this isn't that day. These aren't the right conditions. This isn't fair to the book, or to me. I put it down and grab my insurance book – the comfort read I'd crammed into the bottom of my bag, just in case.

French Relations by Fiona Walker is a story of love triangles, boozy parties, and bad behaviour. After ten pages, I've forgotten about mosquitos and ice cream. I'm barely aware that I'm on the beach. And I'm starting to realise that, while I'm glad that I challenge myself and I'll always try to get out of my comfort zone, I'm also glad that I have a comfort zone to return to.

There are no bad books or bad readers. There are books for all moods, spaces, and seasons. And I'm so lucky that I get to read them all.

Quitters sometimes win

I often have this conversation with You're Booked guests – and You're Booked listeners. 'If you're reading a book and not enjoying it, when are you allowed to give up? Are you allowed to give up?' I've asked these questions and I've tried to answer them. I don't have any good answers. I can't think of a book that I've given up on entirely. But there are plenty that I've put down and never managed to pick up again.

Director John Waters pointed me towards some advice from author and librarian Nancy Pearl. 'If you're fifty years old or younger, give every book about fifty pages before you decide to commit yourself to reading it, or give up. Over fifty? Subtract your age from 100 and use that as your guide.'[2]

It's complicated. On the one hand, we all know that quitters never win, reading is supposed to be good for us, and if we don't finish Hardy's *The Return of the Native*, no matter how much we loathe it, we're never going to pass our English exams. On the other hand, I always want to argue for pleasure to come first, most, loudest, and longest. If you were made to finish a plate of cabbage when you were a child, you probably vowed, as an adult, that you'd never eat cabbage again. I don't think books are any different. If you've ever felt forced to finish a book you truly hated, it will have damaged your relationship with reading for ever. How can you trust books and believe that they will bring you joy when the sight of a particular cover can still unleash a twist of dread in the pit of your stomach, some years after Sunday night was homework night?

Literary critic Sarah Shaffi wrote, 'It's taken me decades to get to the point where I can start a book, realise I'm not liking it, and then just stop reading it.' She also realised that 'Nothing bad will happen if you don't finish a book you don't like... Not getting to the end of a book doesn't mean you're not clever or emotionally intelligent. It's not a sign of any inadequacies in you, it's just a sign that that book is not for you.'[3]

Reading has taught me to trust my taste and listen to my instincts. However, it's also brought me focus and patience. Essentially, the more I read, the better I am at deciding that it's time to stop reading and whether a story isn't for me – but I'm also better at detecting when a novel might not grab me straight away, but it's about to get good.

If you want to read to reduce your feelings of anxiety, it's important that you let yourself quit as many books as you need to, as often as you like. Especially if reading has made you anxious in the past. You don't need a good reason. I've stopped because a character has reminded me of a very irritating old colleague I haven't seen for a decade. I've put books down because they seemed too long, too short, too slow, too busy. I've stopped reading books because they seemed too sad, and I've stopped reading because a book had too many jokes in it. If you're looking to build a reading habit, you're looking for The One – the book that seems as though it was written *just for you*. Your tastes will evolve, your mileage will vary, and if the books that you've rejected before need to be read by you, they will turn up again. You can change your mind as many times as you like. Every potential outcome is a good outcome. You might find the magical book, which will change your life for the better – but no book is ever going to make your life worse. We choose what we read and all those decisions are reversible. This isn't like getting a fringe.

Challenge accepted

However, there's also an argument for reading through discomfort, boredom and irritation. As a reader, I've learned to show up before I'm ready, and by that I mean, sometimes I pick up the books I'm curious about rather than the books I'm craving. Reading to ease my anxiety has made me a more courageous reader. I know there will always be books I can turn to for comfort and stories where I can reliably find old friends.

In the short term, we can live with anxiety by avoiding it and limiting our contact with anything strange, new, and overwhelming. This makes our days feel safer, but duller. It shrinks our world. Or we can accept that sometimes anxiety will arise. We can increase our tolerance of it, which is difficult, but it might make the world feel bigger. It's easy to stay at home with old friends. It's much harder to go out and attend a party where you don't know anyone. But you might meet your new best friend or the love of your life. And, metaphorically speaking, that's how I met Charles Dickens.

When reading is too hard

Dear reader, may I confess something a little embarrassing? I read *Bleak House* for the very first time in 2022, when I was 37. And I didn't like it very much.

In the UK, we don't simply read Dickens, we *revere* him. (In fact, I suspect a lot of us might be doing more revering than reading.) Most of us are familiar with his stories long before we pick up any of his books. He was a prolific writer and a social reformer, successfully drawing attention to the poor conditions of working-class lives and pushing for change. He shaped the world we live in. Lest we forget, he was also racist, anti-Semitic,[4] and plotted to have his wife, Catherine, put into a lunatic asylum.[5] Still, Dickens is a literary institution and an industry. I live near Broadstairs, in Kent, which is, to all intents and purposes, a Charles Dickens theme park because Dickens went there on holiday a few times. I worry that being a reader and a book lover and *not* loving Dickens is a bit like going to church and volunteering to do the flowers and organise the raffle when you're not that keen on God.

However, it's easy to claim a vague literary connection with Dickens through nothing but the power of osmosis. He's still so continually culturally present that I think we can all *feel* as though we've read him without doing any real reading. One venerable You're Booked guest talked at length about their enormous passion for Dickens and how his work had shaped their own. When I asked them if they had a favourite work, they thought for a minute and said, '*A Christmas Carol*.' Which is (a) wonderful, (b) very short, and (c) a story we all feel *extremely* familiar with, thanks to the Muppets. I adore *The Muppet Christmas Carol*, but I have a feeling I'm not the only person who needs to be reminded that Dickens did not write anything about lighting lamps and not rats.

But my father, a voracious reader, would tell you, quite honestly, that Dickens is his most beloved writer. He's not hiding a Jack Reacher paperback behind his heavy, leather-bound books. Dad studied law and qualified as a barrister, so he's especially fond of anything that explores the vagaries of the British legal system in deep detail, which *Bleak House* does. We've bonded over books for as long as I can remember, which is why it was important for me to try to read a novel that meant so much to him.

I knew it was going to challenge me, but I hoped the story would distract me from my feelings of anxiety and put many of my fears into perspective. This was a deep and detailed book about deprivation and devastation. If I started my day with *Bleak House* and I was forced to consider the conditions in which some Londoners lived in the 19th century, I was hardly going to worry about what would happen when I got up and checked my emails.

Training and preparation

In some ways, I believe that every single book I've ever read trained me to read *Bleak House*. Reading for pure, happy pleasure gave me the energy and impetus to pick up a challenging novel. I don't believe that Dickens is 'better' than my favourite authors. In my opinion, Marian Keyes has contributed just as much in terms of social reform,[6] and she's much, much funnier. But the more I read and the more I gained from my reading habit, the less intimidated I felt by a book that had always seemed dauntingly heavy.

When a new Marian Keyes novel comes out, I don't have to make time to read it. I make time to do other things, like showering, eating, and talking to my husband. But I realised that if I was ever going to read Dickens as an adult, it would require some scheduling. If I could find 15 minutes a day for *Bleak House*, I'd finish it eventually. And, if nothing else, it would absolve me of the vague sense of guilt, resentment, and unfinished homework I had whenever I found myself in Broadstairs.

For about a month, I read two chapters of *Bleak House* as soon as I woke up in the morning. At first, progress felt slow – the book seemed tiring. My mind wandered and I often had to go back and reread the paragraph I'd just read. But, after a week, I started to fall into the novel. Instead of waking up and thinking 'Oh, no, I have to read Dickens!' I felt curious and I looked forward to reading another instalment of the story (which was how it was originally read – as a monthly serial). Limiting myself to two chapters meant that I never felt overwhelmed. When I was finding Esther exceptionally irritating, which was often, I just had to get to the end of the second chapter and try again the next day.

Struggling

I was shocked when I realised how difficult it was for me to pay sustained attention to and digest the meaning of what I was reading, especially with the Dickens. My mind wandered. I didn't know what was going on and I felt confused, angry, and alienated. This was the serial that enthralled readers across society! The whole point of Dickens is that he's not just for the wealthy, educated, or 'well-read'! He's *supposed* to be for everyone! As I was struggling, that must mean I'm stupid.

If I'd followed my instincts, I would have given up. But, as I kept trying and felt my focus returning, I started to find confidence, even joy, in my project. It reminded me of being an early reader and realising that, if I just kept practising, and kept getting a little bit better, soon I'd be able to read anything I wanted. The moment reading starts to come more easily to us, we take it for granted. When we read something that feels 'difficult', we can rediscover that old, thrilling feeling of slowly mastering a vital skill.

The act of trying, struggling, and trying again reminded me that our learning is never static. The experience of reading an old book put me in touch with a brand-new feeling. I was capable of changing and expanding. And if I could sit with the discomfort I felt when I was trying to understand this difficult book, I could sit with other kinds of discomfort too. And I might discover something magical when I came out the other side.

I didn't enjoy *Bleak House*, but I didn't regret my time with Dickens. I was grateful for it. I felt proud of myself. I'd completed a challenging project and I'd changed, as a writer and as a reader. Even though I hadn't always found the task easy or enjoyable, I'd stuck with the assignment, and I felt stronger and more capable for it. And sometimes, it *had* been enjoyable. The moments of pleasure and connection weren't instant, but when they came, they felt good because I'd earned them. As a reader, I'd stepped out of my comfort zone. This didn't mean that I couldn't return to the books that made me feel soft and warm, but it meant that, in the future, my reading wouldn't just be defined by my craving for comfort; sometimes I could let my curiosity lead the way.

Happy habits

My focus on Dickens' words first thing carried through and was sustained all day. I felt more present and better at paying attention to one thing at a time. This was evidenced by a lot of smaller habit changes. If I was waiting in a queue at the supermarket or post office, I didn't immediately get my phone out, to distract myself. I think I became a better listener, which made me a better podcast host but, more importantly, a better friend, sister, and partner. And when it came to work – interviewing authors for the podcast and for live events – I felt stronger and more confident. When guests listed the books they'd read and loved, I didn't feel embarrassed by my ignorance or the holes in my own reading. I felt excited to try the 'difficult' books they loved rather than intimidated by the reader and their choices. Overall, I felt less anxious and more capable of dealing with my anxiety when it arose.

Reading Dickens meant I became part of a conversation that has been taking place among authors for nearly 200 years. I'd learned something new about storytelling, sustaining subplots, creating characters, and maintaining tension. Noticing my strong responses to different parts of the story made me think hard about what gives a book life and pace, and what makes a reader want to read. I have no doubt that reading *Bleak House* has made me a better writer.

It might even be fun

Right now, I'm reading *Middlemarch*. This is another book that seemed vast, dry, and intimidating. A book I didn't read because I didn't have time, because other, newer books needed my attention, and because I was embarrassed that I hadn't already read it. Better, smarter people than me said they loved it. What if I didn't? What would that mean?

Several people had recommended it to me, including one of my favourite writers of all time, Jilly Cooper. Both women are readers and writers, and both are fans of beauty and plot. Cooper's books are the ones I pick up when I'm in the greatest need of comfort and I'm desperate for escapism, fantasy, and fun. It was Cooper's endorsement of *Middlemarch* that gave me pause. If she loved it, surely it wasn't going to be a dusty love story about people plodding around their respective parishes? Maybe it might be… *fun*?

It is fun! As with *Bleak House*, it took me a little while to connect with the rhythm of the book. Sometimes my mind wanders, and I need to skip back and reread passages about electoral reform or old town feuds. But it's entertaining, it's funny, and it's filled with characters I can love, and love to hate. In nearly every chapter, George Eliot makes a shockingly prescient observation. Her line, 'People are almost always better than their neighbours think they are', could have been written about life today.

Stolen attention

I don't think I'd be reading *Middlemarch* if I hadn't read *Bleak House*. And I wouldn't have read *Bleak House* if I hadn't read the complete works of Marian Keyes, and Nancy Mitford, and every single other author who made reading fun for me. Many of us meet Dickens for the first time when we're at school – a place where, sadly, reading for pleasure is rarely a priority. We can't pay attention when we feel that our attention is being stolen. We can't cultivate any confidence in our reading when we're told that something is good and good for us – and we're made to feel that if we don't like it, we're in the wrong.

Reading is always subjective. I believe reading fiction when we're young is vital because it helps us to find out who we are – and much of that comes from finding out what makes us feel excited and what makes us feel bored, alienated, or annoyed. When we find something that we love in a book, and something we connect with deeply, we feel vulnerable. It's difficult to express that vulnerability in a classroom.

The best thing about books is that they wait for us, until we're ready to read them. They're patient. Please don't feel guilty about not reading *Bleak House*, or *Middlemarch*, Marian Keyes, or Jilly Cooper. But maybe in a year, or ten years' time, you'll see *Middlemarch* in a charity shop or someone will mention it on the radio, and you'll remember reading this and be curious enough to pick it up and try.

The other wonderful thing about books is that they don't need us to love them. They want to move us, teach us, and entertain us. But they don't require anything from us, apart from our attention in the moment. If we love them, they will stay with us for ever. But if we don't, they won't hold it against us.

Your reading habit is defined entirely by you. This book isn't a trick – I haven't been briefed by an old teacher with a grudge to fool you into reading *Bleak House* or *Middlemarch*. And I don't think that reading either book makes me any more 'well read' than someone who is embarking on their 14th reread of *Elmer*. However, I believe that reading 'big' books can lead to big gains. They require a relatively small investment from us: all they need is a little time and a lot of concentration.

Scary books and self-doubt

So many of us doubt ourselves, our knowledge, and our experience, even though we have every right to be confident about those things. We call our expertise into question. We invite people to contradict us and we don't put ourselves forward for anything unless we're more than sure that we can deliver it. We're put off 'big books' because we feel intimidated by them. We worry that they're for clever people, not us. We think the people who choose to read those books are better and smarter than we are.

The only difference between us and those 'other' people is the books themselves. When you read any 'classic' book – whatever that word means to you – you'll discover that you're just as good as every other person who has ever read that book. The 'big' book now belongs to you, for ever. You can be confident in your intelligence and your opinions. In essence, nothing has changed; you have as much right to speak up as you ever did. But you might find that, as you become a braver reader, you become braver in real life. You stop being afraid of everyone who ever made you feel stupid because you know you're smarter than that.

Reading 'big' books has made me a more patient person. I'm not in such a hurry for gratification and I'm not continually disappointed when nothing works instantly. From new friendships, to trains, to my broadband connection, I'm much better than I was at staying positive and waiting to see what will happen. I've realised that I waste the most time when I'm trying to save it. It's easy to rush around, abandoning projects and people when we realise they're less than perfect – and we find we don't sustain connections or finish what we started. Especially because we have so much choice, we think things will be better somewhere else, with someone else.

In teaching myself to read the stories that scare me, I've taught myself not to run away as soon as a situation starts to feel difficult or displeasing. I've learned to take books, and life, one chapter at a time. And I've discovered that hard books feel harder when I worry about if and when I'll ever finish them and I start trying to calculate how long it will take me to get to the end – which I do with any intimidating project. But I've learned that it's fine to go slowly, so long as we keep going. It might be really hard to find an extra five minutes for a book that has become boring, but we'll never regret reading one more chapter.

I believe this is why books are magical. Some stories rush up to meet us and seem to deliver everything we need from them instantly. If it wasn't for those stories, there's no way I'd be a reader. They make reading feel effortless and I think reading needs to feel effortless. Life is difficult and demanding, and reading should be a refuge from those demands, not another test to pass or fail.

However, I also believe there's a place for the books that challenge us, the books that don't welcome us in straight away. These books have so much to teach us. The rewards come more slowly, but they're worth waiting for. These books make me proud to be a reader and excited about the even bigger books that might be waiting for me in the future. Who knows how much I'll learn, grow, and change?

Creating – and curating – the comfort zone

While we can learn a lot from 'big' books, there's another side to the reading story. We find the energy to reach for the books that challenge us by drawing strength from the ones that feel soft, familiar, cosy, and safe. My dad may be the biggest Dickens fan I know, but *Bleak House* isn't his only favourite book. Every Christmas, he picks up *In the Fifth at Malory Towers* by Enid Blyton.

It's a festive classic. The fifth-formers are asked to organise the Christmas entertainment for the whole school and the story is full of, to use J. B. Priestley's phrase, 'cosy planning'. My dad read it for the very first time when he was 11 or 12, having 'borrowed' (stolen) it from his big sister. And I know that his rereading is a delicious, satisfying tradition for him because he loves the Malory Towers universe so much. Even when he was reading the book for the very first time, the story felt familiar because he'd spent so much time with these characters.

Without giving too much away, there's some very satisfying character development. Vulnerable characters discover hidden strengths. The most thrillingly obnoxious characters start to become self-aware. There's a new girl, Moira, who is satisfyingly awful – and readers are united with the other pupils in their loathing of her – plus there's one of Blyton's greatest comic set pieces of all time, French mistress Mam'selle's 'treek' (dated phonetic spelling and xenophobic stereotyping Blyton's own).

But why does my (now retired) father still derive so much pleasure and joy from reading a book that he almost knows off by heart? Why do so many people read the Harry Potter books from start to finish then, as soon as they've shut *Deathly Hallows*, pick up *The Philosopher's Stone* and start all over again? (I've heard rumours that Margot Robbie is reading Harry Potter on a perpetual loop.) Why do I read *Rivals* by Jilly Cooper every December?

Self-soothing
Even those of us who consider ourselves to be voracious readers – perhaps *especially* those of us who read a lot – will admit to ignoring a pile of new, unread books occasionally, so that we may

reach for something loved and known. We do this even though we often also feel that we 'should' read more and we want to read more. Some people think rereading 'doesn't count'. Asha, 34, says, 'My comfort read is *The Hunger Games*. If I'm posting a photo of everything I've read in the last month, I'm not going to include *The Hunger Games*. It would be quite embarrassing if people saw how regularly it popped up! Not because it's YA – it just feels like a different experience from my other reading. There's something about rereading that feels incredibly intimate to me. I think it's because it's so soothing. That book lives in my head and my heart and sharing a picture of it on social would be almost like posting a selfie where I was sucking my thumb.'

Asha's words make sense to me. Occasionally I struggle with insomnia and, when it strikes, I lull myself back to sleep with one of Sophie Kinsella's Shopaholic books. These novels are comic masterpieces and I'm not embarrassed about loving them or reading them regularly. But I don't always mention them when a friend asks me what I'm currently reading because they're too precious to me for critical discussion. These are the stories I reach for when I'm feeling vulnerable and need to self-soothe or when I'm yearning for a sense of safety. Reading is, by far, the healthiest coping mechanism I have. Perhaps if we all spoke more openly about comfort reading and rereading, more people would discover that books are a mental health resource.

Why it's good for us

Finding comfort in a familiar story might deliver short-term release and relief, but it's also boosting brain activity and deepening comprehension of the book. Rereading definitely counts as reading. The charity BookTrust found that, in adults, 'the re-experience allows them not only to refresh their memory of the past experience, but the recollection is accompanied by the discovery of new details. Therefore, the experience is different, even though it is repeated. By doing it again, people get more out of it.'[8] Perhaps, the first time we read a book, we're desperate to process the main events and key information as quickly as we can. Then, when we return to it, we can start to understand *how* a story is told.

For me, rereading feels like being in on a secret. I'm able to pick up on hints and clues and retrace the path the author has led me down. Rereading has made me a more active, thoughtful first-time reader too. I'm better at paying close attention to the details that enhance a story, so I engage with the story more actively. I'm participating in a different way, responding to the words rather than simply expecting to be entertained. That's not to say there's anything wrong with reading purely for entertainment – it's a completely valid way to connect with the text. Rereading has shown me that there are many ways to experience the same story. You get a lot of bang for your book.

A form of time travel

When the world seems overwhelming and uncertain, it's incredibly reassuring to know that you can keep returning to a corner of it in which everything stays the same, and the experiences you enjoyed previously are there waiting for you too. When friends have been experiencing a 'reading block', struggling to pick up books and pay attention, I suggest returning to a childhood favourite. It's a form of time travel. It returns us to a point in our lives when we had more time and space. It helps us to make room in our heads to imagine and dream.

This is why I reread *Ballet Shoes* at least once a year. Every time I pick it up, I can successfully block all thoughts of mortgages, deadlines, and dinner plans from my head. It makes me eight years old again, and I'm very keen to stay in touch with my eight-year-old self. She was a dreamer and a problem solver. She could be impatient for change, but was an optimist. She thought about the future all the time and was excited about it. And if she'd known that in 30 years, she'd be a grown-up lady who was allowed to read and write whatever she wanted, whenever she wanted, she would have been *thrilled*.

When we pick up a book from our past, we get a chance to befriend our younger self and show them how far we've come. When you're feeling raw and ragged from anxiety, this can be a nourishing, healing balm. Your past self isn't worried about the worst that can happen. They're in awe of the fact that you have a job/dog/car/can eat chips whenever you feel like it.

The power of play

When I was a child, reading was a crucial part of play. My sisters and I would act out our favourite stories, adding details and embellishments. I daydreamed about being friends with Beezus and Ramona, climbing up the Magic Faraway Tree, or going to the Dew Drop Inn with the Ruggles from *The Family from One End Street*. For most children, playing games is instinctive. We don't say, 'Ah, playtime, this is a vital part of my emotional development and essential to creative growth. To the sandpit!' We improvise. We pick a premise, we assign characters to one another, and we get on with it.

It's only as adults that we understand lifelong play is linked to happiness, resilience, flexibility, and strong mental health.[9] However, it's difficult to sustain a playful spirit throughout our lives, especially when we're prone to anxious thoughts. During an acute period of anxiety, I listened to an interview with professor and researcher Brené Brown, who was speaking about positive ways to lean in to our vulnerability. She revealed that a major theme had emerged during her research: play is vital for all of us, at every age. Brown added, 'I noticed in my research that wholehearted people – my term for men and women with the courage to be vulnerable and live their lives "all in" – shared something else, too: They goofed off... Wholehearted adults *play*.'[10] I was horrified. How could I play? When would I play? I tried to imagine myself attempting a game of musical bumps. Immediately, I felt self-conscious and scared – completely estranged from all that was loose, joyous, and carefree. I couldn't play; I'd be bad at it.

But I started to think about the way I played when I was a child. I didn't enjoy games with rules or ones that reward participants for being the fastest or strongest. The games I loved were the ones that you made up as you went along, where you collaborated and created an evolving universe. This is exactly what happens when we read fiction. Whenever I read a book that I loved as a child, I was connecting to the part of myself who played in that way. The girl who didn't worry about being good or bad, but loved being carried away by the sheer power of her imagination.

Brown explained, 'Play – doing things just because they're fun and not because they'll help achieve a goal – is vital to human development.'[11] Having fun is critical to our wellbeing. This is the greatest argument for rereading that I know. If you enjoy returning to a loved, familiar story, you'll know that nothing else matters. You're not unlocking an achievement, tackling your TBR pile, or completing a project. You're finding a way to play and reconnecting with the version of yourself that made play a priority. I believe comfort reading and rereading stokes a fire that fuels our capacity for play. When I feel anxious, reading a beloved old book like *Ballet Shoes* distracts me from my most acute worries, gives me comfort, and calms me. But I believe the long-term benefits are even bigger. Once I'm soothed and safe, I have a stronger foundation to plan, dream, and play.

How to find your reading comfort zone – and finding the strength to venture out of it

Timing is everything. I've learned, when I'm trying to read a book that seems difficult and daunting, I need to start with short, sharp bursts of concentration. If I read for 10 or 15 minutes at a time, early in the day when I have more mental energy, I find that the story starts to stimulate and engage me.

I keep 'comfort books' for moments when I'm feeling energetically and emotionally low. I don't have to work to find my way into the story, I can just let it hold me.

If you can find a way to make a 'hard' book feel easier, embrace it. Watching a screen adaptation might enhance your understanding of the story. Listening to it as an audiobook might make it feel more accessible.

Most of my comfort books are on my Kindle, which means I can reach for them when I wake up in the middle of the night and need to read to get myself back to sleep. I've adjusted the accessibility settings, and I read light print on a dark background, with no backlight, so it doesn't wake my husband up!

I also put my comfort first. My relationship with reading is so precious to me, I can't afford to compromise it by reading too many 'hard' books. Regularly turning to an established 'comfort canon' fuels my passion for reading. This means that, most of the time, I'm then excited about picking up a challenging book. But if life is feeling overwhelming or if I'm more anxious than usual, comfort wins. I need to trust that reading will deliver everything I need from it. There are times when life is daunting enough – we have plenty of other challenges – so we don't need books to become another one.

'Have you reread any good books lately?' Some comfort rereading

Ralph's Party by Lisa Jewell

I first read this late 90s smash hit in the year 2000, when I was 15. I've just reread the 25th anniversary edition. Revisiting this sharp, funny love story reminded me of a time when I was desperate to begin my grown-up life and looking for as many clues as I could find about what contemporary adulthood was like. To me, *Ralph's Party* still reads as the ultimate evocation of fun, sophisticated

London living. It's dense with detail – spliffs, home-made curries, international supermarkets, art openings, Soho sex shops, affairs, designer clothes, staying up all night – and, best of all, true love based on genuine friendship. When I interviewed Lisa Jewell on 'You're Booked', she told me that one of the books that inspired *Ralph's Party*, and defined her view of cool, fun London living, was *The Colour of Memory* by Geoff Dyer. I read it, loved it, and now it's one of my comfort books too.

American Wife by Curtis Sittenfeld

Every time I go back to this book, I discover something new. Sittenfeld's imagined version of Laura Bush's life story is written with warmth, curiosity, and clarity. Alice, the school librarian turned First Lady, is written in such a smart, sympathetic, and endearing way that I feel as though I'm spending time with one of my kindest and cleverest old friends every time I'm reunited with her. The novel doesn't shy away from complexities and contradictions. It's frank about the pain of grief and the way we must live with our biggest mistakes. But it always absorbs any big feelings I bring to it. It builds a world that forgives its inhabitants for not finding instant, straightforward solutions. And it elevates the importance of empathy – a quality that always loosens the grip that my anxiety has on me.

Postcards from the Edge by Carrie Fisher

Fisher's very funny debut novel is the perfect cure for all feelings of nebulous dread. When I'm overwhelmed by those weird waves of guilt, horror, and anxiety that don't seem to have any obvious root, I turn to this story. It's about actor Suzanne Vale and the array of people she meets at rehab – including the obnoxious, delusional Alex, who will reassure any insecure reader that their life is not a total disaster. Having a bad day? Did you spend thousands and thousands of dollars on cocaine, then drop it in the bath? No? You're doing fine.

11
Reading
for
COURAGE

"Scared is what you're feeling. Brave is what you're doing"

Emma Donoghue[1]

I lean against the wall and try to do the breathing exercise I saw on YouTube. In for four. Hold for four. Out for four. This is just adrenaline. It's a good thing. It shows how much I care. It would be weird if I wasn't terrified.

In, two, three, four... it isn't working. Have my lungs shrunk?

I look at my phone. I just need to get through the next four hours. Four lots of 60 minutes. I try to list all the four-hour chunks I've endured over time. The waitressing jobs I've had – running around, being shouted at by stressed-out chefs for spilling things. At least I don't have to spend the next four hours wearing socks soaked with gravy. I don't have to sit a maths exam. I don't have food poisoning. Surely, I'd rather be here, by the Guildhall in London, immobilised by fright, than sweating and vomiting on my bathroom floor?

Although, if I did have food poisoning, I'd have a very good excuse for getting out of this. My stomach is definitely on some kind of spin cycle.

About a month ago, I received a very exciting phone call from a producer at the BBC. Would I join the news team, live, at the Booker Prize ceremony as a guest presenter when the winner was announced? I was stunned, flattered, and thrilled. I said 'yes' straight away. It sounded like an extraordinary opportunity. My gut knew it would be terrifying when the time came, but if I did everything my gut told me to do, I wouldn't do anything. I'd never leave the house. And my ego loves to write enormous confidence cheques, so long as they're dated quite far in the future. But right now, I'm in no position to cash any of them.

I've prepared as carefully as I can. I've read every book on the shortlist. I thought I'd done the most terrifying part of the work – reading Lucy Ellman's 1,000 page, one-sentence novel, *Ducks, Newburyport*. It was described to me as a postmodern masterpiece, and I was terrified that I wouldn't get it. But I fell in love with its hypnotic rhythms, its slow, exquisite rendering of the dramatic and domestic, love, terror, and doom. And I was already familiar with some of the books. I'd been lucky enough to pick up a proof copy of Bernadine Evaristo's vivacious, electric *Girl, Woman, Other*, which was far and away my favourite. But what if my opinions are all wrong? And I was bound to muddle dates and names. What if someone asks me to analyse the seminal moment on page 47 of Salman Rushdie's novel? I'm going to be sick.

The bricks behind me don't feel solid. I'm reaching for support, but my fingertips are clawing at the air. I can't do this. I know nerves. I know anxiety. But this is different. I think my body is shutting down in protest. And I can't make anyone understand because I'm always doing things like this. I say 'yes', every time I'm asked, so that's why I think no one believes me when I tell them I'm terrified. I remember an old schoolfriend whose severe lactose intolerance was no match for her addiction to ice cream. That's me. That's what I'm doing.

But I don't have a choice. I've got to dig deep and find the courage to leave the wall and walk to the Guildhall.

Ducks, Newburyport is a book about anxiety. A story about what it is like to churn with fear about the slow collapse of civilisation while working, running a home, and tending to your children. And *Girl, Woman, Other* is about many kinds of fear. The fear of the unknown, and the other, is what keeps your world small. I think about Evaristo's character, Carole, and the violence and abuse she endured – and the alienation she felt when she arrived at university. She wanted to run. She returned. I think about Penelope, whose racism and prejudice is rooted in fear. I've been captivated by these characters. I've been dazzled by the talent and courage of their authors. They have been truly brave. All I have to do right now is walk for five minutes and be in a building for four hours.

Maybe I'll say something stupid on live TV. Maybe I'll fluff something, panic, or become tongue-tied. But how will I feel at the end of the night? If I go home now, I'll be ashamed of myself. The instant relief will give way to self-loathing and regret. But if I step into the fear and allow it to consume me, I know it will end. It might go wrong. I might do this badly. But it has to be better than not doing it at all.

I take a step forward, and another, and another. The fear is powerful and muscular, forcing its weight against my chest, clinging to my back, pushing my shoulders down. It's coming with me to the Guildhall. Even though I definitely don't get to bring a plus one. But, as I carry it and focus on stepping and breathing, stepping and breathing, I know that I'm doing the right thing. Next time – there will be a next time – this unwieldy animal will feel a little bit lighter. And, maybe one day, it will simply weave itself around my legs before releasing me to my duties. I've got to feel weak if I'm going to get strong.

Fear is inevitable

Working for the BBC on the night of the Booker Prize remains one of my proudest achievements. Not because of the prestige of the gig – or even because I did a good job – but because I turned up. I experienced one of the most acute anxiety attacks that I've ever felt as an adult. And I didn't let it win. I understood how to work with my fear. I stepped into it and embraced it.

It has taken me a long time to understand that fear is an inevitable part of life. It's easy to avoid it, up to a point. We can arrange our days and schedules to ensure that we almost never have to leave our comfort zones. But what happens when fear eventually, inevitably catches us – and we don't have the tools or resources to deal with it? And are there ways that we can become more courageous?

Fear, anxiety, and bravery

I believe 21st-century courage has been defined by education activist Malala Yousafzai. In October 2012, aged 15, she survived an assassination attempt by Taliban gunmen. She was returning from an exam. At the time, the Pakistani Taliban had banned girls from attending school. Her activism started when she was just 11. She started writing a blog for the BBC about living in Swat, a district where the Taliban were gaining a foothold. Other students refused the assignment because it was so dangerous. She wrote about what it was like to see her school shrinking and to see her friends missing their education because of the fear the Taliban instilled in everyone. More than 100 schools were blown up in Swat before the education ban became official. Malala risked her life every day she attended class.

On her 16th birthday, Malala gave a speech at the United Nations. 'The terrorists thought they would change our aims and stop our ambitions but nothing changed in my life except this: weakness, fear and hopelessness died. Strength, power and courage was born.'[2]

Almost none of us will ever know what it's like to live in a war zone or to risk our lives for our education – and the education of our peers. But we can all be inspired by Malala, her work, and her words. It's easy for us to assume that her courage is innate, that she's changed the world through her fearlessness. But her speech shows that this isn't true. 'Weakness, fear and hopelessness' were present within her, as they are, sometimes, in all of us. Her bravery didn't come first; her courage was forged by fear.

Courage is being able to do something even though it frightens us. Fear and bravery are both completely subjective. I don't need to dig *too* deep into mine to catch and release a spider. It's not my favourite activity, but I'm not being brave when I manage to get it into a glass before sending it back out into the wild. For my arachnophobic sister, though, this is a feat on a par with going into a lion enclosure and giving the residents a dental check. Bravery doesn't come naturally – if it does, it isn't bravery.

Standing up and speaking out

We have seen another compelling example of 21st-century bravery in climate activist Greta Thunberg. Aged 15, she started a series of climate strikes, refusing to attend school until her home country of Sweden reached compliance with the Paris Climate Agreement. Thunberg is autistic and has been diagnosed with selective mutism – an anxiety disorder that makes speech impossible in triggering situations. What she's done is awe-inspiring. Many of us struggle to stand up, speak out, and draw attention to ourselves in small-scale situations. But Thunberg, who is living with an anxiety disorder so acute that it stops her speech entirely, still manages to address the world. She's *not* fearless – she speaks because she's prioritised another kind of fear. 'I want to feel safe. How can I feel safe when I know we are in the greatest crisis in human history?' she wrote in an essay published in Swedish newspaper *Svenska Dagbladet*.[3]

Yousafzai and Thunberg both started their activism when they were remarkably young. Many of us have been startled by their maturity, intelligence, and grace. We remember being teenagers, worrying about exams, and feeling unable to string a sentence together. We assume that courage comes from experience, not youth. I always believed that I'd feel braver as I got older, but a 2015 University of Haifa study found that fear tends to *increase* with age. Young rats were able to eliminate fear in their brain quickly, but adult rats retained the fear, even after the triggering event had passed. And, in humans, our fear response is connected to our developing prefrontal cortex and amygdala. Our response is more variable, but the less flexibility and plasticity we have in our brain – which decreases with age – the more fear we tend to feel.[4]

Fear and action

I think that our changing attitude to bravery might be influenced by the different messages we hear as children and adults. Even as an easily frightened child, I understood that without bravery, nothing could be done. The world was a daunting place, filled with difficulty, but we all had a responsibility to meet that difficulty head on and accept any challenges that came our way. In the stories I read, I learned that if you were put in a position which required you to take on a challenging task, it meant the adventure was about to begin.

In Enid Blyton's Famous Five novels, fear – or, at least, showing it – is a moral issue. Bravery is a value and no one really cares how you feel or whether you're nervous or anxious. You're supposed to swallow your emotions and get on with the serious business of solving crimes. In the Famous Five universe, adults are absent or not entirely trustworthy. No one is coming to save you.

Even in 1947, when the first Famous Five book was published, no one would have encouraged their children to take their dog to a deserted island and go to foil some baddies for the sake of developing some vital life skills. But Blyton suggested to her readers that 'having adventures' was a perfectly valid thing to do in the school holidays. I don't think anyone is going to make a case for most of her attitudes and values, but I'm grateful for her stories and the way they celebrated bravery. Yes, it was frustrating when Anne's logical fear responses were dismissed because she was a girl. (For me, it was also frustrating that George was so desperate to dismiss her girlhood, although I suspect that it was important to young gender non-conforming readers to see a character they could connect with.) But Anne, and George, were still included in the story. Girls could be as brave as boys – even if the boys disputed this every step of the way.

Brave books

We don't have to go back to the Famous Five to reconnect with our bravest selves. But when we read stories about bravery, we can remind ourselves of its value and understand that fear is all part of the adventure. In real life, fear and anxiety make me feel isolated. When I step through those feelings, into courage, I need to find a way to rely on myself. But, in fiction, we find plenty of comrades – and the bravest heroes and heroines are usually helped by a supporting cast.

My sister says, 'I reckon I learned everything I needed to know about bravery from the Harry Potter books. A lot of the specific scenarios are fantastical. Hopefully, I'm never going to need to fight any dementors. But, as a young reader, they taught me so much about confidence, power, and standing up for myself. I think the biggest message is that we're never alone. Sometimes, asking for help is the bravest thing we can do, and the best way to summon strength. Of course Harry has unusual, unique gifts, but I wouldn't want to read a story that was just about Harry, using magic to fight evil. Readers love Hogwarts because we all feel as though we could be brave if we went to school there. As an adult, I know that all frightening tasks feel a little more achievable if I'm surrounded by people who believe in me and want the best for me. And, just as importantly, if I'm able to help someone else be brave, I've got to do it, whether that means giving some practical support or an emotional boost.'

She adds, 'I loved *The Lord of the Rings* for that reason too. Any quest is better with friends. When we have to be brave, I think we worry about failure and what can go wrong. If I try and fail as part of a group, I can be sad and disappointed, but I don't feel isolated or ashamed because I have people to share the experience with.'

My bravest book

When I was growing up, my bravest book was – and still is – *When Hitler Stole Pink Rabbit*, Judith Kerr's semi-autobiographical novel about fleeing Germany and becoming a refugee when she was nine. At the beginning, the protagonist, Anna, takes the train from Germany to Switzerland with her mother and elder brother, Max. During the journey, Anna reads a book about the lives of famous, notable people and feels a little left out when she learns that they have all had a 'difficult childhood'. Anna feels that, so far, her childhood has been far too easy to give her a shot at fame and success. Of course, her childhood immediately becomes difficult as the family moves across war-torn Europe.

Talking about her own experiences, Kerr said, 'My parents were wonderful. My brother Michael and I knew there wasn't much money but it didn't seem to matter much. They made us feel it was an adventure.'[5] The book taught me that bravery might just be a question of perspective and attitude. If the story was about Anna and her family continually contemplating the bleak global horror that was on the brink of subsuming everything, the book – and their lives – would be very different. But for Anna and her family, bravery is fuelled by curiosity. They are at their happiest, and most confident, when they let go of all their expectations and find something new and novel in their situation.

Dread and terror lurk in the background, but Anna finds that the only way to live with fear is to seek joy alongside it. Occasionally, she thinks of her old house and her old life and imagines Hitler breaking in and playing with Pink Rabbit, the toy she left behind. But she's quick to acknowledge that no good can come from comparing her old reality with her new one. Anna's attitude allows her to be brave in surprising ways. She's squeamish about eating a snail in Paris on Bastille Day, but she's delighted to discover it tastes like 'a delicious mushroom'. One of her lowest moments comes when she starts school in Paris and she can't understand her teachers, classmates, or lessons. She feels confused, alienated, and exhausted – until, one day, everything clicks. After weeks of immersion, she can understand French.

I love *When Hitler Stole Pink Rabbit* because it's a story of sustained bravery. It's about making a habit out of courage and it reminds me that even during moments of unfathomable crisis, meals must be made, clothes must be washed, and routines must be observed. Kerr makes it clear that Anna and Max are protected by their parents as a matter of duty. Understandably, Anna's mother frays under the strain of the situation and experiences anxiety and depression. Kerr's message isn't simply that any obstacle can be overcome with a positive mental attitude. I believe she's suggesting that we can help ourselves to tap into our innate bravery if we're prepared to seek out as much joy as we can. When I'm faced with a challenge, I still ask myself what Anna would do, how Anna would find a way to persevere. And, as I get older, I think of Mama, Anna's mother. If I can't summon the resources to be brave for myself, maybe I can be brave for my husband, or my sisters, or my friends.

As young readers, we can relate to stories in which characters are called on to act in brave bursts because childhood requires a lot of courage. We're asked to meet the unknown every day. Our fears change over time. I'm not sure when I became scared of parties or stopped being afraid of the dark. Books put me back in touch with all the different ways in which I've learned to be brave. They remind me of what is possible – with or without magical powers, money, difficult childhoods, or gangs of orcs to defeat. Without fear, there is no bravery. And without bravery, there is no story.

How we can all be a little bit braver

- **Ask for help** When you're feeling overwhelmed by the task in front of you, try to find someone who can hold the ladder, figuratively or literally. Look for a friend whose skills complement yours. If that's a struggle, speak to someone who can say, 'You got this!' *and mean it*. Ideally, someone who has known you for a while and will say, 'I know you're scared about the presentation, but do you remember how nervous you were before the Nativity play? And you smashed it! You were the best innkeeper Mrs Howman had ever seen!'
- **Make the project into a quest** You have the skills for this, and identifying and gathering the right team is a skill in itself. To be brave, you have to be honest with yourself about your strengths – and what you're good at as well as about what scares

you. Think about the Famous Five. Every single member of the gang had a part to play. You might be a Julian, with vision. You might be an Anne, bringing a necessary note of caution. Bravery doesn't always mean acting alone and, with the right team, you'll discover just how brave you can be. (Hopefully, you're not Uncle Quentin.)

- **Embrace curiosity and novelty** We fear the unknown because we're worried that it will harm us, but it might just turn out to be our new favourite thing. We can build up our bravery muscles by seeking out new experiences, like Anna in *When Hitler Stole Pink Rabbit*. Think of the first time you tasted oysters, mussels, or olives. Or the first time you visited a brand-new city, on your own. Make a list of the times that facing a fear has rewarded you and get into the habit of trying out new things as often as you can. When the stakes are higher and you've got to step up and do something scary, you'll feel prepared, positive, even excited. (I've had to train myself to become a more adventurous eater. Every time I feel a bit nervous about a new dish, I tell myself that I'm using my mussels muscle.)

More brave books

The List of Suspicious Things by Jennie Godfrey

Hyper-observant 12-year-old Miv and her best friend, Sharon, want to solve a serious crime. The Yorkshire Ripper is murdering young women and the adults around them are secretive – and scared. Miv is frightened, too, but she believes that she has a responsibility to work out what's going on. This tender, heart-filling story is about emotional bravery and finding strength in friendship. I adored it.

Fearless by Trinny Woodall

If anyone knows anything about bravery, it's Trinny. This is a book about everything she's learned in her life and her career – from addiction and rehab to building a business. I think she proves that curiosity is the cure for fear. She still isn't fearless, but she invites us to fear less. And she's excellent at finding small ways to feel brave and making sure they stack up.

Here Again Now by Okechuckwu Nzelu

This beautiful book contains layers of love stories. It's about grief, passion, and heartbreak, but it deftly explores the fear that lives behind hate. Ekene's world is shattered when his closest friend and sometimes lover Achike dies suddenly. But he forges a tender relationship with Achike's father – a man who has to come to terms with his homophobia and understands the way fear has shaped the way he lives his life. It's a book that reminds us the less we fear, the more we love.

12
Reading around
THE WORLD

"Reading makes immigrants of us all. It takes us away from home, but more important, it finds homes for us everywhere"

Jean Rhys[1]

It's early March, 2020. I've just given a talk at the University of Gloucestershire. I spoke about imposter syndrome, perfectionism, and how we get in our own way. Speaking to students about these subjects is important to me because it gives me a chance to share everything I wish I'd known when I was a young adult. That confidence isn't something other people are simply born with, and if you don't feel confident, it doesn't mean you don't have anything to be confident about. That genuine self-belief doesn't come from being focused on the self, but from being curious, generous, and open to learning about the world around you.

On the train home, my imposter syndrome starts to rise up, at the back of my throat. I could choke on it – it's put me off my complimentary packet of shortbread. I can access the whole world through my phone, so I do. I start by scrolling through Twitter (now X). I'm looking for jokes, information, observations – anything that might make me think or laugh. Predictably, most of the messages and conversations are about the coronavirus.

About a month ago, my sister Beth had sent me a link to a news story about the coronavirus. She was scared. Beth has severe health anxiety, which flares up in times of stress. She's very good at finding things to worry about. I made unhelpful suggestions. 'I don't think this is anything we need to worry about. Don't google it.' Secretly, I rolled my eyes.

I'm starting to realise that I owe Beth an apology. Not least because I can't stop googling. Twitter is flooded with strange, dark rumours about warehouse morgues, shortages, and international lockdowns. I go to *The Guardian*'s website, BBC News, the *New York Times* – any news outlet that might be covering the emerging story in a clear-eyed way. (I avoid the MailOnline website, because I know exactly what to expect – WE'RE ALL GOING TO DIE and somehow this is Meghan Markle's fault.)

Only 30 minutes ago, I was standing in front of hundreds of students, telling them everything I've learned about living in the world. Rapidly, it's becoming apparent that I know nothing at all. The apocalypse is approaching. And I've just told a group of smart, ambitious, vulnerable young adults that they can cope with anything if they find ways to develop some self-belief. I dared to suggest that I had some knowledge and experience I could share. Yet, here I am, frowning at my screen, typing in my stupid searches. 'Coronavirus + pandemic over soon?' 'Covid + death.' 'Covid + food shortages.' 'Covid + cure.' My brain ran its own separate, secret searches. Can you die of Covid anxiety? Would I? How can I think so selfishly? How much do I need to know about this?

The breadth and depth of information available seems infinite. The state of the crisis is unknowable because there is so much to know. I wait for one voice of reason to rise up and establish a sense of calm. I look for instructions. Instead, the voices clamour. They are angry and scared and accusatory. Why don't I know enough? Why can't I do more? Why does nobody know what will happen?

Glimpses of the globe

When I was growing up, I thought journalism was one of the most important jobs that existed. It held the keys to understanding the world and our place in it. In the early 90s, I saw glimpses of the Gulf War and the famine ravaging Somalia on the early evening news. I was awestruck by the reporters. They put themselves in the most frightening situations imaginable but were able to speak about what they saw with sombre clarity. It seemed like a thrilling, fascinating, dangerous way to live. And I felt grateful for their courage. It seemed important that everyone should know what was happening everywhere. There would be no way of knowing what the news was if it weren't for the people who risked their lives to report it.

But news was worthy. It was serious. It could be bleak. It wasn't supposed to be tawdry, scandalous, or gripping. I was vaguely aware of tabloid newspapers and their covers – the disconnect between *The Sun*'s 'paedo panic' and their promise of teenage 'stunnas' on Page 3. I remember thinking it was weird that they seemed to invent their own news cycle. One year, they were fixated on killer Rottweilers, the next they demonised 'asylum seekers' – a phrase that confused me as I associated it with Quasimodo and Esmeralda seeking sanctuary in *The Hunchback of Notre-Dame*. How could anyone possibly object to helping a vulnerable person who needs protection?

Most of all, I noticed the contrast between the red, dramatic newspapers I saw in shops – all capital letters, exclamation marks, sex, violence, and panic – and the boring newspapers that my dad brought home. Lots of pictures of elderly white men on the front and headlines like 'Reform bill proposed'. It didn't occur to me that knowing as much as you could about what was happening could be anything but useful. Or that information could be addictive.

The medium is the message

At university, I became involved with student journalism. I fell in love with writing features. My colleagues would seek out serious stories; I was interested in trends, people, and how we were living. After I graduated, I ended up on the Features desk of teen magazine *Bliss*. I adored my job and took it very seriously indeed. For our readers, an exclusive interview with One Direction was every bit as important as a 'Reform bill proposed' story.

When I started working as a journalist, the world was different. News came from newspapers, television, and magazines. The idea that you'd read the news on your phone, or a blog or Facebook post might include a credible news source would have been laughable. Over the next few years, the way we wrote news and the way we responded to it changed completely.

Now, we're overwhelmed by information – and many of us want to read in a different way. In the quest to ease our anxiety, it may be time to read less and understand more. If you think that bingeing on information makes you feel worse, don't worry. There's a way to read widely and understand more about the world that will help you to feel informed, empowered, and confident enough to make changes.

News junkies

In 2020, the *Oxford English Dictionary* made 'doomscrolling' a word of the year, adding it to the dictionary and defining it as 'the action of compulsively scrolling through social media or news feeds which relate bad news'.[2] The word was coined by journalist Karen K. Ho in response to the volume of news content we have near constant access to, which is overwhelming. Ho recognised that many of us struggle to cope with it. At the start of the pandemic, as a public service, she started to tweet reminders intended to interrupt the doomscrolling flow. These were simple suggestions, telling followers to stretch, go to bed, or drink some water. It seems so obvious, but it shows how a news addiction can grip us and how difficult it is to stop scrolling when your hunger for information is insatiable. 'What doomscrolling does is rob future you of the energy you need to really focus on important things,' Ho told *Scientific American*.[3] This is the issue that so many of us have. We scroll because we care. We want to stay informed, but when we take in so much information, we become overwhelmed. We're drained of the energy we need to preserve if we want to make a difference.

Nothing ever changes

It comforts me to discover that doomscrolling is a new word for an existing problem. Communications professor Dr George Gernber created the term 'mean world syndrome'[4] to explain the impact exposure to news can have on our cognitive bias, which is that it causes us to see the world as more dangerous than it actually is. Under normal circumstances, we can contextualise the news as part of the lives we're living. Often, although the news is distressing and upsetting, when we're regularly seeing people we like and love, we don't feel so exposed to the worst of the world. The 'mean' stuff has a context, and we hear positive, hyperlocal news too. Pregnancies, engagements, promotions. And stories that may seem trivial, but are incredibly important to our wellbeing – funny anecdotes, weird things a nephew said, new recipes attempted. Book recommendations. During the various lockdowns, we couldn't exchange this news in person and, because normal life was suspended, we also had fewer opportunities to create good news. There was therefore generally less of it to go around. As a result, and because there was simply more of it anyway, bad news made up a greater percentage of all news than usual. Mean world syndrome had more space and it thrived.

Serious stress

Our bad habits did not help. Before Covid, we had been glued to our phones to find out as much as we could about Brexit and Trump – and the endless reports of global and local injustice. So, by 2020, most of us were already burned out by bad news. Many friends told me that they were feeling more anxious than they'd ever been. One, another journalist, said her news addiction was causing her so much stress that she'd started to grind her teeth in her sleep. 'There's never a moment to process what's happening, because everything seems to change by the hour – and it's always getting worse,' she said. If you're an anxious person with a news habit, it's hard to shut off the news completely – especially when your body and brain seem to be telling you that finding out new information is the only way you can survive.

After the first lockdown was announced, I decided to limit my news intake. The worst-case scenario had happened and all I could do was follow the rules. It became apparent that the news wasn't *new*. The information we were receiving was being repackaged, embellished, and repointed. But I wasn't learning anything. I was simply receiving instructions telling me how to feel. Every headline I read seemed emotive, written to generate feelings of anger or terror. So I started to avoid the news as much as I could.

However, this position became untenable. In May 2020, George Floyd was murdered by Derek Chauvin, a police officer, in Minneapolis, Minnesota. Protests and marches were organised across the world and Floyd's death sparked a global conversation about racism, responsibility, and how to be a better ally. This was news that could not be avoided. It was distressing and upsetting. But we had to engage with it as a matter of urgency. Our lack of engagement was part of the problem.

Some friends suggested that we organise a remote reading group. Together, we discussed Layla F. Saad's book *Me and White Supremacy*, working through the journaling exercises and vowing to be as honest as we could with one another about the ways it was challenging us. It was a difficult and necessary experience. I'm so grateful for Saad's words and work, and for the friends who came together and made us all accountable.

At the time, the conversation about racism and privilege on social media was deafening. There was a lot of noise, confusion, and performance. Many writers, speakers, and creators, including Saad, were generously creating resources and sharing them on social media, but I found it difficult to focus on those resources or to understand them in a meaningful way. Everyone seemed to be reacting quickly and shouting over everyone else. Reading

Saad's book felt like entering a quiet room and being granted the space to give her prose the attention and respect it deserves.

Dysregulation

When I watch rolling news coverage for too long, I feel dysregulated. I'm overwhelmed, overstimulated, and then I crash, as though I've eaten a lot of sugar. I have the same empty, nauseous, wired feeling – having consumed something with no fibre, no context, and no nutritional value. Reading a book like Saad's gives me context for the news. The situations she's describing are no less urgent than the ones I'm seeing on TV or online, but her words allow me to understand the issues in the context of the wider world. They force me to unpick my unconscious bias and lazy tendencies.

On social media, the news is an unstoppable force, hitting me in waves and happening *to* me. When I read more deeply, the news becomes my responsibility and I start to understand how I can act and why I need to act. Saad forces her readers to question their white fragility.

Before I read her book, the news made me feel anxious, ashamed, and guilty. After I read her book, I felt less anxious and more confident, purely because I was better informed. She made the point that it is better to be proactive and risk making a mistake and being called out than it is to stay silent. Social media had made me cowardly. I'd grown up idolising the brave journalists who stepped into their fear and spoke out. I needed to reconnect with that part of myself.

Reading for context

I wasn't the only person who found solace and sense in books when trying to navigate the news cycle. Book sales increased sharply in 2020[5] and, at the start of the pandemic, there was a surge of interest in a particular classic backlist title – Albert Camus' 1947 novel *The Plague*.[6]

The novel is loosely based on the 1849 cholera epidemic following the French colonisation of Algeria, where Camus was born. It's an absurdist novel – Camus writing from the point of view of the universe being meaningless, so when we look for meaning in the world, we come into conflict with it. 'What's true of all the evils in the world is true of plague as well. It helps men to rise above themselves', Camus wrote. 'There is more to admire in humans than there is to scorn.'[7]

Some readers looked to *The Plague* to find parallels between the situation in the fictional town of Oran and the global pandemic and lockdown life in 2020. I think I learned more about our situation from Camus' novel, than I would have done from the news. In *The Plague*, people in positions of power are slow to respond to the seriousness of the situation. Everyone is wracked with fear and anxiety, and the unknown future seems much darker and more daunting than the present disaster. The situation seems to bring out the best and worst in people, and as Camus concludes, goodness prevails.

Initially, I was reluctant to read the book. We were living through a real-life plague. I didn't understand why anyone would want to immerse themselves in a fictional one, for fun. But Camus' book broadened my perspective. It filled me with gratitude, which is a wonderful balm for anxiety. The people of Oran struggle to obtain basic resources and can't take simple hygiene for granted. I was locked down in a flat where I could take a bath whenever I wanted. Having to queue outside the supermarket for toilet roll was no hardship – especially when I usually ended up buying Toblerone too.

Most importantly, *The Plague* forced me to understand that the world has always been, and will always be, vulnerable to unprecedented events. I started to reconsider my anxiety. It made me very focused on myself. Subconsciously, I believed it was down to me to keep the worst at bay. I suspected there was a bizarre butterfly effect at play and if I missed a deadline, skipped a gym visit, or forgot to reply to an email, everything would start to unravel. The collapse into chaos would be my fault. The message of *The Plague* made me embrace my own powerlessness, in an empowering way. I concluded that the energy I expended on worrying could probably be put to better use.

Empowering reading

Shortly after reading *The Plague*, I read Abi Daré's acclaimed debut, *The Girl with the Louding Voice*. I fell in love with Adunni, the teenage heroine who longs to become a teacher. She bravely escapes her arranged marriage to pursue her dreams. Around that time, my friend Hilary introduced me to an organisation called Kiva, which supplies loans to unbanked people across the world, helping women to set up businesses and become economically independent. Since I've signed up to Kiva, I've invested in several projects, including a farm in Nigeria, a solar-powered freezer distribution company in Uganda, and a woman-led dairy in Kenya.

Daré's novel takes an unpalatable truth – the abuse of girls and women in Nigeria and the economic pressure on their families – and tells the story of one of these girls in a hopeful way. It's fictional, but it has truth at its core. This is a situation that rarely gets the news coverage it deserves. In novel form, as readers, we're forced to consider it and absorb it – we can't skim it in the way we might the front page of a newspaper. Most importantly, Adunni's courage is inspiring. Her story isn't tragic, and the novel made me feel as though taking any action would be worthwhile. For me, that meant supporting organisations like Kiva and mentoring young women closer to home.

How to help

Another lockdown book I loved was *You People* by Nikita Lalwani – a novel about a London restaurant, staffed mostly by undocumented chefs and waiters, and Tuli, the proprietor, who is doing his very best to protect and support the vulnerable people he has employed, sometimes in unorthodox ways. This is a book about how a whole world can be found within a city, about the stories we all carry, what it means to offer refuge, and how to build a life. The story is told through the eyes of Nia, who has fled an alcoholic mother in Wales, and Shan, a Tamil refugee who has left a young family behind in Sri Lanka.

Lalwani's prose is beautiful, and this book is a pleasure to read, but I loved it most for its measured, considered exploration of an issue that is rarely discussed with any sense of calm or nuance. It's a book that dares to suggest immigration is a problem with no easy answer, and it's impossible to fully untangle the chains that trap the most vulnerable people in society. I told a friend about the book and she told me about her work mentoring with the Kent Refugee Action Network. They're always looking for donations and support (at the moment, they're asking for people to help fund bikes, lights, and road safety courses for the people they work with. I just bought a helmet!)

Perhaps it sounds simplistic, but I believe that reading about the world can prompt us to understand it and to change it for the better. To put it another way, when I'm online and I learn about a crisis or a disaster, I feel powerless and overwhelmed. My emotions are unmanageable and I feel guilty and ashamed about the fact that I'm even considering my painful feelings when I should be supporting the people who are directly affected by the crisis. When I try to find out how to help, there's usually a chorus of contradictory voices, shouting about how all our efforts are wrong and, ultimately, pointless.

But when I read the work of writers like Lalwani, Daré, and even Camus, I can only think about the real people and real situations that exist beyond their novels, and I feel inspired and energised. The authors draw my attention to the facts beyond the fiction and they call me to act.

What my podcast guests suggest

Talking to guests on You're Booked, I realise I'm not alone. Many of us feel confused and overwhelmed when we're trying to stay informed, so we've turned to books to get a greater sense of the state of the world and our place in it.

'One book that really helped me during the first part of 2020 was Adam Gopnik's *A Thousand Small Sanities: The moral adventure of liberalism*,' Adam Buxton told me, during a recording of You're Booked.[8] 'At a time when everything felt extreme and heightened, it explored what was going on in the world in a sober, thoughtful way. And it pointed me towards other great, useful books too. I discovered the work of Bryechan Carey, Harriet Taylor Mill, and Michel de Montaigne. Montaigne's essays seemed startlingly contemporary. He made me realise that nothing we worry about is really that new.'

Josie Long revealed that reading renews and refreshes her sense of optimism and helps her to focus on the positive and the possible. 'One book I'd recommend is *From What Is to What If: Unleashing the power of imagination to create the future we want* by Rob Hopkins,' she said. 'It's about the power of play and imagination, and how it's vital to nurture our imagination if we want to make the world better. It's very difficult to be creative when you're waiting for the worst to happen. This book looks at the activism that might be possible when you release yourself from some of that anxiety.'[9] Emma Dabiri recommended *A Thousand Plateaus*, a book by philosopher Gilles Deleuze and psychoanalyst Félix Guattari, both working in France, which explores philosophy, maths, and capitalism in a post-structuralist, postmodernist way.[10] There's something very sobering about trying to see big changes and social anxiety through an academic lens.

'If we share a story, our minds move along the same tracks and occupy the same imaginary landscape, and this can bring us together'

If anyone understands the benefits of reading widely and becoming wiser, it's author and TED speaker Ann Morgan. In her book *Reading the World: Confessions of a literary explorer*, she writes about undertaking an enormous project in 2012 – reading a book from every single country in the world, which is the 196 different territories recognised by the United Nations (UN). I wanted to ask Ann how her project had broadened her perspective – and whether it had changed her or made her braver.

I interviewed Ann for this book just after her trip to Assam, where she had been teaching reading workshops. 'These are my Incomprehension Workshops. I started them because I realised that the way we're taught to read has such an impact on our reading. We need to do a kind of unlearning. In my *Reading the World* project, I discovered that I had so many unexamined prejudices, in terms of what I expect from books and people. I wanted to teach these workshops to get people to notice when they feel uncomfortable with a book – and to find ways to sit with that discomfort, instead of putting the book down. What can we learn about our own cultural conditioning, when we start to explore what makes us feel uneasy?'

Ann said that she's often asked whether she discovered a universal aspect of storytelling when she was reading the world. 'Everything I read was very different, but the project showed me that the act of storytelling itself is universal,' she said. 'The fact that everyone loves to share stories is the force that bridges so many divides. I draw a lot of strength from that – no matter where people are, and what challenges they face, they want to tell stories about their experiences, and I think that's a very hopeful thing.'

I was expecting Ann to tell me that reading so widely showed her how much we have in common. However, she said one of the best things about the project is it's taught her that our differences can be cherished and celebrated. 'I have extraordinary interactions with people who are so different to me in so many ways. I've talked about sex with a Mormon reader in the US, I've had a correspondence with a schoolboy in Afghanistan. Stories give us common ground. Even if we look at the world very differently, if we share a story, our minds move along the same tracks and occupy the same imaginary landscape, and this can bring us together.'

This is heartening, especially at a time when our differences seem alienating and polarising. 'When I spend time on social media, I notice that people seem so focused on spotting and weaponising their differences,' I told Ann. 'Especially when we're talking about what's going on in the world.'

Ann said, 'We tend to imagine that news is fairly neutral and objective. But of course, it isn't. It's a story that's told with certain agendas. We might imagine it's opening our eyes and informing us, but it's just reinforcing what we already think we know about how the world works, and what things are like in different places. Whereas a story that is told from a very different perspective takes you inside that experience and starts to show you how maybe some of the ideas you might have assumed were universal really aren't.'

Ann also believes that we're in a different mental space when we read a book, which gives its message room to permeate. 'A news article can be shaming. We feel as though we're being coerced into urgent action, so we have our guard up. But when we read, we come to the experience with a more open heart. Eventually, we take a richer, more nuanced view of things. That doesn't necessarily always mean that we go out and volunteer for something or give money directly. But it might just change some of the choices we make over time or the role we take in discussions or the opinions that we back, which I think is how meaningful change happens over time. It's about gradual, incremental steps that people can sustain.'

I find Ann's project inspiring, but am a little daunted by the prospect of reading so far beyond my comfort zone. Where can we begin? And what do we do if we're finding reading overwhelming. 'Reading can make us feel better, but on the flip side, we do need to have a certain level of mental quiet in order to engage with a book. To start something like this, we need a bit of equilibrium, and there will be periods of your life that are too turbulent to read something that challenges you. If you're not in a place where you're able to do that, just pay attention to yourself and listen to your responses. Don't beat yourself up. Just trust yourself that it will pass, and you'll find your way to calmer waters.'

Ann said that reading so widely has changed the way she sees the world, but it's also had an impact much closer to home. 'I think reading gives us the keys to ourselves. It was humbling to meet books that didn't necessarily want me to understand them, as well as books that taught me how to read them as I went along. I studied literature at university, and I prided myself on being a "good" reader, learning the context, knowing how a text should be read, and being able to make clever observations about it. But I wasn't able to bring any of that to my year of "reading the world" – and knowing less really opened my eyes to my own habits and conditioning. Best of all, I learned about the generosity of readers. I still can't believe the number of people who helped me by sending me books, and translated text that wasn't available in English, just because they were excited about my project. Their kindness and enthusiasm were truly life-affirming.'

Talking to Ann was exhilarating. It made me realise that we can all read for comfort *and* courage. I hope you're excited about the idea of embracing your discomfort, challenging your prejudices, and discovering what you don't know yet. This is a big step in our reading journey. We don't have to read this way, all the time. But reading for pleasure might be the fuel that gives us the energy to read for perspective too. And the books that change our minds and lives won't necessarily be heavy or difficult. Writers like Daré and Lalwani are taking complicated issues and bringing them to our attention by writing about them with hope and joy. As our minds expand, we'll become more ambitious, curious readers – and we'll find more pleasure in a wider range of books.

Reading around the world: how to broaden your literary horizons

- **Start small** If you'd like to learn about as many different places and hear from as many different voices as possible, short story collections are a great way to begin. You could try the collection by Frank Wynne, *Found in Translation: 100 of the finest short stories ever translated*. See what sparks your curiosity and where these stories lead you.
- **Talk to booksellers** If you go into any independent bookshop, you'll find someone who is happy to recommend a book by a brand-new voice. If you tell them about the other books you enjoy, they'll be able to guide you towards the perfect choice. I know this might sound daunting but, for what it's worth, I've never met a bookseller who didn't love being asked for a recommendation. No one is going to judge you because you're not already familiar with international books. They'll be excited by your interest.
- **Don't be afraid of the obvious** You might want to read a classic, like *The Plague*, or you might want to start with a writer you've heard of, like Stieg Larsson, Elena Ferrante, or Haruki Murakami. It doesn't matter where you begin, you'll get something from any book you choose. Hopefully, you'll enjoy the book so much, you'll want to keep going.
- **Make yourself uncomfortable** Or, rather, notice when you're reading something and you feel your barriers going up. Every single one of us has an array of unconscious expectations, prejudices, and ideas, no matter how open-minded we try to be. We'll never eliminate them, but reading widely will help us to understand what we assume and what we take for granted.

Books to read to learn about the world
Cause Celeb by Helen Fielding
Fielding's first novel is extremely funny and was ahead of its time. It's a satire about charity, emotional exploitation, and white saviourism. Rosie has her heart broken and flees from London to volunteer at an aid camp in North Africa. When famine looms, she turns to her ex and his celebrity friends to lead the fundraising. This book shows us how to help and be useful by showing us what not to do.

My Brilliant Friend by Elena Ferrante
The first of Ferrante's acclaimed Neapolitan novels is the story of friendship, but it's also about class, poverty, and opportunity. Ferrante writes about the way education brings down walls, yet money and the absence of money can shrink our worlds. It opened my eyes to unseen injustices and the ways that women are still trapped by tradition.

Women Talking by Miriam Toews
This book was inspired by real life events. Between 2005 and 2009, in the Manitoba County Mennonite colony in Bolivia, more than 100 girls and women were gassed and raped in their sleep. Toews writes about the secret meetings between the eight Mennonite women who have 48 hours to decide what to do in response. The novel makes us look at something that we'd rather not see. It gives victims faces and voices, and forces us to attempt to comprehend the incomprehensible. It's unexpectedly irreverent in places too. It's a story of horror and shared humanity.

Epilogue
Turning the page

"Unlike in the movies, there is no THE END sign flashing at the end of books"

Elif Shafak[1]

My reading habit hasn't cured me of anxiety. It's done so much more for me than that. It's made life deep and rich. It's given me the ability to look upwards, and outwards. It's taken me out of myself and given me a way to be by myself. It's made me realise that I cannot count my blessings because they're infinite. On my darkest, most difficult days, it's shown me that I don't need to be ashamed of any of my feelings because they have all been felt before. And it's helped me to find a safe way of examining those feelings and holding them up to the light. It's shown me that nothing and no one is entirely strange. We are all different and we are all the same. We are all optimistic, overwhelmed, helpless, bold, grandiose, frustrated, well-intentioned, petty, loving, horny, self-conscious, marvellous messes. We can't escape ourselves, in Beirut or Blackpool. We can never fully know ourselves or one another. But we can know one another better with every book we read.

And reading itself creates a refuge. The world can be a noisy, flashing, chaotic assault on the senses, which leaves us dysregulated and alienated. My reading ritual provides a restorative shelter, protection against the overwhelm. It brings me connection when I feel estranged. It engages my mind in a way that makes it easier to live in my body. It guides me to find focus when I feel distracted. When I feel crushed by the pressure to be purposeful and productive, it gives me the space to play.

As Ann Morgan (author of *Reading the World*) says, reading gives us the keys to ourselves. I think the worst thing about anxiety is the lies it tells us. It turns us into confused strangers and makes us forget all that we can do, all that we are. My anxiety is shaped by my low self-esteem. My brain will come up with a vague, nebulous problem and, even before I understand what the problem is, I feel as though there's no way to fix it. But, as a reader, I have answers. All books are helpful manuals, detailing all the vague, nebulous problems that humanity has ever faced, from war strategies to difficult job interviews. I can look my anxiety in the eye and tell it that I know the answer – and if it isn't on the tip of my tongue, I can find it somewhere on my bookshelves.

I hope you're excited about building your reading habit and watching it evolve. We've talked about how reading can help us to learn and grow. We've explored the ways in which reading can make us kinder, braver, calmer, and funnier. But it's time for you to begin the next phase of your reading journey – and that might feel daunting. While books can ease our anxiety, the anxiety itself builds barriers. It can make it very difficult for us to sit still and focus on something beyond ourselves. After all, you're never alone when you have a relentlessly critical inner voice!

When I was at my lowest ebb, I hated being alone with my thoughts so much that showering was an ordeal. I felt worthless. At the time, I thought my feelings were proof that I was 'bad' at my job. Every morning, as soon as I woke up, before I was fully conscious, I started listing the reasons for my incompetence and the colleagues who disliked me the most. I felt like a frightened child. I didn't know that I had any control over the situation. I didn't think of myself as an adult who could choose how she regarded herself. I didn't know I could choose to value myself. Every day, I waited for something good to happen – for someone else to approve of me and neutralise the emotional acid building up within me. Of course, this never happened – because I was carrying out a self-fulfilling prophecy. I was setting myself up to fail, thanks to cognitive bias. I could only see evidence of my 'badness'. I don't think I'd have noticed if my boss lit up fireworks inside the office, spelling out the words, 'GOOD JOB, DAISY'.

Eventually, my anxiety became so unmanageable that my GP offered to sign me off work. That's when I decided to leave my job. I knew myself well enough to realise that sick leave would probably make me even sicker, the dread of the return building and building. And, as soon as I came to this conclusion, I started to gain a little more perspective. My anxiety didn't end, but it lifted a little. It stopped pinning me to the ground. Before I could start to read my way out of it, I had to take remedial action. Here's the very first thing I did. It's trite, it's twee, and it's the sort of act that's beyond parody. If you've ever rolled your eyes at someone's Instagram affirmations, you will roll your eyes at this. But it saved me. It helped me to start putting myself back together.

I edited my phone alarm, so I was woken up by this reminder: 'BE KIND TO YOURSELF!!!!!!!!!!' And if I had the time, resources, and access to some sturdy ladders, I would have spent my mornings travelling all over the country, knocking on your windows, beseeching you to do the same, because I'm a reformed cynic when it comes to kindness.

I've made many mistakes. I've tried to earn kindness. I've tried to prove myself worthy of it. I've tried to trick people into giving it to me. It's only through getting to know my anxiety, and myself, that I've learned anything about how kindness works. You can call it empathy if that feels a little less cloying, but it's our fuel. It's the fire that lights us up, keeps us warm, and we need to keep stoking it. We can't ever afford to let it burn out. If we can find ways to fill ourselves up with it, we'll always have plenty to spare.

Anxiety thrives when there is an absence of kindness. I'll always have some anxiety, but kindness stops the anxiety from defining me. Would things change for you if I promised you that, no matter what you did, or didn't do, you are worthy of love, respect, encouragement, patience, play, and rest? What would it take for you to believe that?

We can't read when we hate ourselves because hate doesn't allow much room for anything beyond self-obsession. We can't concentrate when every word seems to contain an affront or assault. My reading habit has made me more compassionate, inside and out. But I needed to start with love, to make sure that books did not become another stick to beat myself with.

This is why I like to read in the morning – it's a way to start the day with love. It has changed the way I feel about myself. It means that I don't start by listing all the things that are wrong with me and all the things I need to achieve in the next 12 hours to be a person of worth. It means that I begin with gentle curiosity and play. I'm not proving anything to myself or anyone else. I can lose myself, in the most grounding way. I've learned how my anxiety works. After sleep, my brain tends to rouse itself by shouting, 'WHAT DID WE MISS IN THE NIGHT? WHAT DO WE NEED TO BE AFRAID OF?' If I pick up a book or my e-reader, I can direct its nervous energy. It craves information, so I give it information. It wants to know what's going wrong and what it should be worrying about, so this morning, I let it worry about a burglary in Hannah Dolby's excellent *How to Solve Murders Like a Lady*.

Sometimes I describe anxiety as 'What if?' disease. We, the anxious, have vivid imaginations. We wake up in the middle of the night, on holiday, picturing plugged-in hair straighteners, flames leaping from exploding irons, our front doors wide open and banging in the breeze. We can write grim, bleak, verbose speeches for our bosses within seconds after being tapped on the shoulder and hearing the words 'Quick chat?' (Our anxious brains are a thousand times faster than ChatGPT.) Give us an unexpectedly high electricity bill and we become instant estate agents, moving ourselves out of our homes immediately. 'My problem is that I just can't bear uncertainty,' I once told my therapist. Kindly, she replied, 'Yes, that's an issue for all humans.' We tell ourselves wild, dramatic, hyperbolic stories all the time.

Reading stories that other people have written can give us some respite from our own dramas. And stories remind us that life is sometimes terrible and often wonderful. We're all struggling with uncertainty. And whether we're fictional or real, we're all faced with problems that seem impossible at first – and then we discover that we're capable of solving them.

Best of all, reading can cure us of our addiction to destinations and endings. When my anxiety has been at its most acute, I've believed that I can achieve my way out of it – and then become frustrated when this doesn't work. (It never works.) We can never complete reading. And being a reader has taught me to rest. I've realised that if I force myself to complete all my 'important' chores and tasks before I pick up a book, I won't read a word. But if I make time to read, I can approach these tasks with greater energy, joy, and pragmatism. I'm better at being 'good enough'.

I need to protect my reading and make sure it never becomes a chore. This isn't always easy because there's a significant overlap between reading for work and reading for pleasure. I've said that elsewhere in this book. To maintain my relationship with reading, I must prioritise pleasure. Reading is too precious; I can't afford to let myself resent it. I urge you to do the same, especially when you're building your reading habit. You deserve to be moved, engaged, and entertained. Only read what you love in the moment. And expect the moment to change. The book that leaves you bored and alienated this year might enchant you next year. Your perspective will shift every season, and your self-knowledge and capacity for pleasure will increase.

Readers are my people. Readers are in touch with the magical and the universal. We ask the best questions – and we understand that these are often the most obvious questions. We understand that what we don't know is much more interesting than what we do know. We love details, but we're quick to lift our heads, look up and understand that we're neither the best nor the worst. Reading is what cures us of the conviction that we might be 'a piece of shit that the universe revolves around,' as Anthony Kiedis put it in his memoir, *Scar Tissue*. We're optimists. We believe that the next book we open might be the best yet.

Most of all, readers are not afraid of being alone. We know what to do when we feel lonely and we're happy to be on our own. Because we understand that we're never entirely alone.

It's difficult to be still. It's hard to open yourself to someone else's imagination when your own makes your life hard and heavy. Sometimes, simply starting a story requires courage. But I hope you will try. I believe that the next time you pick up a book, you'll find a balm for your roughest edges. When my anxiety seems to be burning through my bones, reading makes me feel soft but strong. Even if books simply soothe and comfort you, then a reading habit is worth cultivating. But reading won't just ease your anxiety – it will show you the possibilities of a life beyond it. Words will take you to gorgeous, glittering places. Reading will remind you how good it feels to dream. I don't know where books will take you, but I'm so excited for you – and for all of us. From now, anything is possible. Let the adventures commence!

Books that bring joy

Explore these reading recommendations from some of my favourite authors. Here are the books that always make them feel better.

Sam Baker, author of *The Shift*
Ultimately, I land on pretty much anything by Marian Keyes. Despite the fact that her books are Trojan Horses of tough stuff, I know for a fact I've never read one of her books without laughing out loud in inappropriate places. They give me solace. They make me feel safe. They make me feel understood. They make me cry laughing.

Lauren Bravo, author of *Probably Nothing*
I love *Bridget Jones: The edge of reason* by Helen Fielding. Much has been made of Bridget's flaws over the years, but still not nearly enough of her flawless wit and wisdom. I first discovered her aged 14, at a time when romance felt as remote as Jupiter, but my whole world was filled with hilarious, clever girls being joyfully stupid together, and she has been a precious point of connection with so many hilarious, clever, joyfully stupid women ever since (this book's author very much included). I've returned to Bridget countless times over the years whenever I need to fill my cup – this, my favourite of the series, was the comfort book I took to hospital when I gave birth – and many lines are seared directly onto my brain in such a way that it's sometimes hard to tell where my own voice ends and Helen Fielding's genius begins. She's a cultural touchstone, and a personal origin story. V.v. good.

Kat Brown, author and editor of *No One Talks About This Stuff*
If I'm feeling really bad, I reach for extremes of disaster and comfort. *Miss Pettigrew Lives for a Day* by Winifred Watson, *Eleanor Oliphant is Completely Fine* by Gail Honeyman, and *Sorrow and Bliss* by Meg Mason offer the exact balance of catastrophe, tragedy, and redemption that I need when I'm not sure everything will be all right, but I'm willing to suspend that belief for a while.

Charlie Connelly, author of *Attention All Shipping*
My book of joy is *Pinocchio* by Carlo Collodi. When we were kids, my sister and I would spend most weekends at our grandparents' house. Our nan would put us to bed, proper blankets tucked in so tightly as to leave us effectively mummified, then she would read to us. It was always *Pinocchio* and every week she would start from the beginning. This meant that we never progressed past the first couple of chapters, always interspersed with roars to my grandfather downstairs to 'Turn that bleedin' telly dahn'. To this day, I can probably recite the opening pages from memory, but have no idea what happens after Mr Antonio gives Geppetto a piece of wood. Don't want to know. Haven't even seen the film. Those wispy memories are magical enough, thanks very much.

Fearne Cotton, author of *Scripted*
For me, reading is sanity-saving – I don't know what I'd do without books. I prefer to read new stuff, but there are a couple of books that have been lifesaving. One is *The Four Agreements* by Don Miguel Ruiz. It's a beautiful book about esoteric thinking. When I've been at my absolute lowest, I'll come back to that. Sometimes I'll pick a page at random and start reading. At a time when I felt awful, it lifted me up a level and brought me out of the darkness.

Nell Frizzell, author of *Cuckoo*
When I was 23, I went on holiday with a group of three friends I'd had since we started wearing hair mascara and butterfly hairclips in our

early teens. It was the holiday where we discovered a local wine co-operative (nicknamed 'The Cave') where you could simply refill any receptacle with wine from one of the six taps. By day four we were bringing empty olive oil bottles and pouring away our shampoo to make more room. I *may* have at one point just brought a mug. Anyway, we all brought our own books – *To the Lighthouse, A Visit from the Goon Squad, Midnight's Children* – and yet we all, like moths to a flame, eventually gave up these books entirely and, in turn, read a single book found on the holiday cottage's shelf: *Spilling the Beans* by Clarissa Dickson Wright. As we fried ourselves under the French sun, *Spilling the Beans* would go round and we would each in turn be howling or gasping with joy at the next revelation – Clarissa punching an Alsatian dog out cold, Clarissa giving herself a tropical illness from drinking so much gin and tonic, Clarissa having a near-death experience from an underwired bra. It is such an unlikely and brilliant memoir and we still talk about it to this day. I have never, once, watched her show or cooked one of her recipes. Because, for me, Clarissa Dickson Wright isn't a chef or a Fat Lady; she is a literary genius.

Harriett Gilbert, host of *A Good Read*, Radio 4
My creased, yellowing copy of *Cold Comfort Farm* by Stella Gibbons dates from when a paperback cost 35p. It's a glorious novel. Over the years, I must have read it half a dozen times, and every time it makes me happy – in part because Flora Poste's reorganising of her relatives' lives is genuinely laugh-out-loud funny; in part because the book has one of the strangest, most romantic, and beautiful endings in literature.

Jennie Godfrey, author of *The List of Suspicious Things*
I so desperately want to choose a *The Complete Works of Jane Austen* as a book that brings me joy but, if I had to choose just one, it would be *Persuasion*. From romance, to comedy, to social commentary, to drama and pathos, IT. HAS. EVERYTHING. And it's the book I return to again and again if I am ever sad, anxious, or

just simply in a reading slump. Jane's novels can get a bad rap for being narrow/one-dimensional, especially to our modern sensibilities, but I think she captures the imperfection of humans and the human experience beautifully.

Andrew Hunter Murray, author of *A Beginners' Guide to Breaking and Entering*
The Meaning of Liff – I read this as a teenager and it's stayed with me ever since. Douglas Adams and John Lloyd's dictionary of 'things there should be words for', mixed with all the wonderful place names that, until now, have just been loafing around on signposts, is a cult classic. It introduced me to the delights of Swanage, the risks of Glossops, and the enormous relief of a Godalming. I will carry these made-up definitions in my head for the rest of my life.

Robin Ince, author of *Bibliomaniac*
When I have insomnia and I can't sleep, I turn to *The Country Girls* by Edna O'Brien. A more recent book would be *Foster* by Claire Keegan, and I think *Leonard and Hungry Paul* by Rónán Hession would be on that list too. Joy isn't always the word I'd use to describe these books . . . but there's something about the sheer pleasure I get from marvelling at the craft of these amazing writers. All of these books have moved me.

Marian Keyes, author of *My Favourite Mistake*
Gravity is the Thing by Jaclyn Moriarty is my happy book. Because it's defiantly hopeful, even when the laws of physics try to ruin everything.

Clare Mackintosh, author of *I Let You Go*
Aged 11, I fell in love with the Just William books, and the series remains my happy place more than 35 years later. The stories make me laugh out loud, and Richmal Crompton's creative

approach to the passing of time (William and the Outlaws remain the same age throughout the series, which spans 50 years) makes it feel timeless. I feel the same joy when I open the pages now as I did when I received my very first copy.

Katherine May, author of *Wintering*
Lolly Willowes by Sylvia Townsend Warner made me utterly gleeful the first time I read it. So many people had recommended it and, of course, I'd completely ignored them. When I finally picked it up, I first of all revelled in its acerbic commentary on the life of a 'maiden aunt', but then the whole novel jackknifed into something completely unexpected. How many novels peak with their protagonist scolding Satan himself? It's one of the best books I've ever read about women at midlife, and it's a hundred years old. I now recommend it to everyone.

Nikki May, author of *This Motherless Land*
If I had to pick my most loved book, and that's as hard as choosing a favourite dog, it would be *Station Eleven* by Emily St. John Mandel. I've read this dystopian tale, set in the nightmarish years after the collapse of modern civilisation, at least ten times and it *always* sparks joy. The pandemic (which wiped out 99 per cent of the world's population) is just a backdrop – it's actually about people, art, life, religion, and survival. This wistful, dreamy book reads like poetry, driven by values like beauty and goodness. But what I love most about *Station Eleven* is its hopefulness – even in the bleakest of circumstances, humanity can and will thrive.

David Nicholls, author of *You Are Here*
I always go back to *Franny and Zooey* by J. D. Salinger – that's my comfort book. The final pages are about joy, hope, and why you have to keep going. I read it in a shallow, inspirational way, but I find it really moving. That's always a pleasure for me.

Cathy Rentzenbrink, author of *How to Feel Better*
The Pursuit of Love by Nancy Mitford has got me through many a
dark night. It is whisper light, but with a pleasing underpinning
note of pain. And it's funny! Which is always the thing that helps
me carry on.

Dale Shaw, author of *Painfully British Haikus*
My wife changed my life in many ways – and one of the most
formative ways that she changed me was by introducing me to a
certain kind of book. Novels that, from the outside, don't appear to
have vast amounts in common, but which all contain an indefinable
joy – warmth, attraction, humour, and zest, run through with a sort of
yearning. These are books you just don't want to let go. *Happy All the
Time* by Laurie Colwin is the epitome of this kind of book. So little
happens. And the things that do happen seem so slight. Yet, as you
read, you're always on the edge of happy tears, desperate for more,
compelled to continue. Other books with the same DNA include
Brother of the More Famous Jack (Barbara Trapido), *I Capture the
Castle* (Dodie Smith), *Larry's Party* (Carol Shields), *The Pursuit of
Love* (Nancy Mitford), *My Name is Lucy Barton* (Elizabeth Strout), and
Standard Deviation (Katherine Heiny). It's hard to define precisely
what makes them so special, but every one of these books is a gift.

Nina Stibbe, author of *Went to London, Took the Dog*
I turn to any and all Barbara Pym novels, especially her characters
planning their weekday meals… disagreeing about who should be
served duck, the curate or the dressmaker, and who should make
do with cauliflower cheese.

Ericka Waller, author of *Goodbye Birdie Greenwing*
Anne Tyler's writing always makes me feel joyful, and my very
favourite is *The Accidental Tourist*. Especially the scene with the
siblings inventing the card game that no one but them understands.
It's funny and tender and clever and perfect.

Holly Williams, author of *The Start of Something*
I wouldn't call it 'comfort reading' exactly, but Ali Smith's writing gives me so much mind-expanding joy because I know that anything she's written will reliably get the synapses sparking. So intelligent, yet light and playful with it, formally inventive, but with real heart and wit, and reliably both curious and deeply humane, her books make my insides crackle with excitement at what words can do. When I grow up, I want to be Ali Smith.

Acknowledgements

Read Yourself Happy is a book that only exists because of the many wonderful readers and writers I've met and worked with throughout my life. Huge thanks to all of them.

First, I'd like to thank my wonderful editor, Elizabeth Neep, whose imagination, energy, and talent have shaped this book, from its inception. Also, J. P. Watson and the Pound Project team, for their generosity, support, and confidence. *Read Yourself Happy* was inspired by my Pound Project book, *Burn Before Reading* (Birmingham: 2022). I'm so grateful to everyone who supported that book, and I really hope you enjoy this one!

Enormous thanks to the team at DK and DK Red – Elise, Esther, Rebecca, Vickie, Helen, Charlotte, Stephanie, and everyone who has worked so hard to bring this to life. Thanks to Michelle Clark for your wisdom and thoroughness! Big thanks to Matt Brown and the team at ID Audio. Thanks to my wonderful agent, Diana Beaumont, for being such an indefatigable and insightful collaborator – and to the teams at Marjacq Scripts and DHH Literary.

Thanks to my fabulous interviewees – Jill Hanney, Becca Caddy, Dr Sophie Mort, Sarah Ellis, Joel Morris, Ruby Rare, Emma Gannon, Catherine Gray, David Nicholls, and Ann Morgan. And thanks to everyone who shared their stories and lent their voices to this project. I'm so very grateful to all of you.

Huge thanks to everyone who has been such a vital part of my reading life, and to everyone who has been so kind, loving, and patient with me when I've struggled. Thanks to every writer who has written words that have filled me with cheer, joy, delight, and understanding. Thanks to everyone who has listened to the You're Booked podcast, and every guest who has shared their reading stories with me.

Most of all, thanks to Dale, who is my all-time favourite writer, reader, and collaborator. I love you more than you know.

Notes

Introduction

1 'Mental health facts and statistics, Mind, n.d., available at: www.mind.org.uk/information-support/types-of-mental-health-problems/mental-health-facts-and-statistics/#:~:text=Specific%20diagnoses&text=Mixed%20anxiety%20and%20depression%3A%208,Depression%3A%203%20in%20100%20people (accessed August 2024).

2 Joe Pindar, 'Anxiety statistics UK: 2023', Champion Health, n.d., available at: https://championhealth.co.uk/insights/anxiety-statistics/#:~:text=In%20any%20given%20week%20in,access%20treatment%20(Mental%20Health%20Foundation (accessed August 2024).

3 John Green, *The Fault in Our Stars* (London: Penguin, 2013).

1. Read yourself calmer

1 Henry Williamson, *Tarka the Otter: His joyful water-life and death in the country of the two rivers* (first published, London and New York: G. P. Putnam's Sons, 1927; London: Puffin, 2014).

2 'Uncertain times: Anxiety in the UK and how to tackle it', Mental Health Foundation, 2023, available at: www.mentalhealth.org.uk/our-work/public-engagement/mental-health-awareness-week/anxiety-report (accessed August 2024).

3 'What is anxiety disorder?', Mental Health UK, n.d., available at: https://mentalhealth-uk.org/help-and-information/conditions/anxiety-disorders/what-is-anxiety/#:~:text=In%20the%20UK%2C%20a%20little,will%20experience%20the%20same%20symptoms (accessed August 2024).

4 Marc-Antoine Crocq, 'A history of anxiety: From Hippocrates to DSM', *Dialogues in Clinical Neuroscience*, September 2015, 17(3), pp. 319–25, available at: www.ncbi.nlm.nih.gov/pmc/

articles/PMC4610616 (accessed August 2024).

5 Zaria Gorvett, 'How the news changes the way we think and behave', BBC Future, 12 May 2020, available at: www.bbc.com/future/article/20200512-how-the-news-changes-the-way-we-think-and-behave (accessed August 2024).

6 Rolf Dobelli, 'News is bad for you – and giving up reading it will make you happier', *The Guardian*, 12 April 2013, available at: www.theguardian.com/media/2013/apr/12/news-is-bad-rolf-dobelli (accessed August 2024).

7 Nikita Gill, 'How to break up with your phone: On hyper-connectivity doing a number on our brains', How to Survive an Existential Crisis, 20 May 2024, available at: https://nikitagill.substack.com/p/how-to-break-up-with-your-phone?utm_source=profile&utm_medium=reader2 (accessed August 2024).

8 'Parasympathetic nervous system (PSNS)', Cleveland Clinic, n.d., available at: https://my.clevelandclinic.org/health/body/23266-parasympathetic-nervous-system-psns (accessed August 2024).

9 Rebecca Gross, 'Why it pays to read', National Endowment for the Arts, 16 January 2015, available at: www.arts.gov/stories/blog/2015/why-it-pays-read (accessed August 2024).

10 Anne Lamott, *Almost Everything: Notes on hope* (Edinburgh: Canongate, 2019).

2. Read yourself secure

1 Roald Dahl, *Matilda*, illustrated by Quentin Blake (London: Puffin, 2022).

2 'Facts and statistics about loneliness', Campaign to End Loneliness, n.d., available at: www.campaigntoendloneliness.org/facts-and-statistics (accessed August 2024).

3 Andrew J. Arnold, Heather Barry Kappes, Eric Klinenberg, and Piotr Winkielman, 'The role of comparison in judgments of loneliness', *Frontiers in Psychology*, 24 March 2021, 12, available at: www.frontiersin.org/journals/psychology/articles/10.3389/fpsyg.2021.498305/full (accessed August 2024).

4 'Social comparison theory', TheoryHub, n.d., available at: https://open.ncl.ac.uk/academic-theories/34/social-comparison-theory (accessed August 2024).

5 Rachel Ehmke, 'How using social media affects teenagers', Child Mind Institute, 24 May 2024, available at: https://childmind.org/article/how-using-social-media-affects-teenagers (accessed August 2024).

6 Rob Newsom and Dr Anis Rehman, 'Sleep and social media', Sleep Doctor, 22 December 2023, available at: www.sleepfoundation.org/how-sleep-works/sleep-and-social-media (accessed August 2024).

7 Julia D. Buckner, Rebecca A. Bernert, Kiara R. Cromer, Thomas E. Joiner, and Norman B. Schmidt, 'Social anxiety and insomnia: The mediating role of depressive symptoms', *International Journal of Depression and Anxiety*, 2008, 25(2), pp. 124–30, available at: https://pubmed.ncbi.nlm.nih.gov/17340615 (accessed August 2024).

8 'The Queen's Reading Room Study', The Queen's Reading Room, 2024, available at: https://thequeensreadingroom.co.uk/the-queens-reading-room-study/#:~:text=Key%20findings%20revealed%20that%20just,feel%20ready%20to%20tackle%20challenges (accessed August 2024).

9 Helen Thomson, 'Why adolescents put themselves first', *NewScientist*, 8 September 2006, available at: www.newscientist.com/article/dn10030-why-adolescents-put-themselves-first (accessed August 2024).

10 Diana I. Tamir, Andrew B. Bricker, David Dodell-Feder, and Jason P. Mitchell, 'Reading fiction and reading minds: The role of simulation in the default network', *Social Cognitive and Affective Neuroscience*, February 2016, 11(2), pp. 215–24, available at: www.ncbi.nlm.nih.gov/pmc/articles/PMC4733342 (accessed August 2024).

11 Helen Fielding, *Bridget Jones's Diary* (London: Picador, 2014).

12 TEDTalks, 'Sarah Ellis and Helen Tupper: The best career path

isn't always a straight line', TED, YouTube, 11 June 2021, available at: www.youtube.com/watch?v=1ALfKWG2nmw (accessed August 2024).

3. Read yourself funnier

1 E. M. Delafield, *Diary of a Provincial Lady* (first published, London: Macmillan, 1930; Pan Macmillan, 2016).
2 Ron Charles, 'Finally, a comic novel gets a Pulitzer Prize', *Washington Post*, 17 April 2018, available at: www. washingtonpost.com/entertainment/books/comic-novels-never-win-the-pulitzer-prize-except-this-year/2018/04/16/cbde8e52-41c6-11e8-8569-26fda6b404c7_story.html (accessed August 2024).
3 Charles, 'Finally, a comic novel gets a Pulitzer Prize'.
4 Helen Lederer, *Not That I'm Bitter* (London: Mirror Books, 2024).
5 'Stress relief from laughter?: It's no joke', Mayo Clinic, 22 September 2023, available at: www.mayoclinic.org/healthy-lifestyle/stress-management/in-depth/stress-relief/art-20044456#:~:text=Laughter%20may%20ease%20pain%20by,you%20connect%20with%20other%20people (accessed August 2024).
6 Dr Paul Wright, 'Your brain on laughter: What happens in your brain when you laugh?', Nuvance Health, 18 September 2022, available at: www.nuvancehealth.org/health-tips-and-news/your-brain-on-laughter (accessed August 2024).

4. Read it and weep

1 E. B. White, *Charlotte's Web* (first published, London: Hamish Hamilton, 1952; London: Puffin, 2014).
2 Sofie Boterberg and Petra Warreyn, 'Making sense of it all: The impact of sensory processing sensitivity on daily functioning of children', *Personality and Individual Differences*, 2016, 92: pp. 80–6, available at: www.researchgate.net/publication/288687054_Making_

sense_of_it_all_The_impact_of_sensory_processing_sensitivity_
on_daily_functioning_of_children (accessed August 2024).

3   Pelagia Horgan, 'Crying while reading through the centuries',
    New Yorker, 3 July 2014, available at: www.newyorker.com/
    books/page-turner/crying-while-reading-through-the-centuries
    (accessed August 2024).

4   Tom Whipple, 'Why is the world getting sadder?: Global survey
    uncovers a worldwide increase in distress and mental health
    struggles', *The Times*, 27 March 2023, available at: www.
    thetimes.co.uk/article/why-is-the-world-getting-sadder-
    9qbtkw83d#:~:text=The%20findings%2C%20from%20the%20
    Gallup,reverted%20to%20the%20previous%20trend   (accessed
    August 2024).

5   Jaber S. Alqahtani, Ahmad S. Almamary, Saeed M. Alghamdi,
    Saleh Komies, Malik Athobiani, Abdulelah M. Aldhahir, and
    Abdallah Y. Naser, 'Effect of the COVID-19 pandemic on
    psychological aspects, in Mohammad Hadi Dhghani, Rama Rao
    Karri, and Sharmili Roy (eds), *COVID-19 and the Sustainable
    Development Goals: Societal influence* (Amsterdam: Elsevier,
    2022), pp. 235–58, available at: www.ncbi.nlm.nih.gov/pmc/
    articles/PMC9334998/#:~:text=conclude%20that%20
    depression%2C%20anxiety%2C%20posttraumatic,pandemic%20
    than%20before%20the%20pandemic (accessed August 2024).

6   Rob Picheta, 'The world is sadder and angrier than ever, major
    study finds', CNN, 25 April 2019, available at: https://edition.
    cnn.com/2019/04/25/health/gallup-world-emotions-index-scli-
    intl/index.html#:~:text=People%20worldwide%20are%20
    sadder%2C%20angrier,Global%20State%20of%20Emotions%20
    report (accessed August 2024).

7   Kavitha Cardoza and Clare Marie Schneider, 'The importance of
    mourning losses (even when they seem small)', NPR, 14 June
    2021, available at: www.npr.org/2021/06/02/1002446604/the-
    importance-of-mourning-losses-even-when-they-seem-small
    (accessed August 2024).

8 Glennon Doyle, *Untamed* (London: Vermilion, 2020).
9 Toketemu Ohwovoriole, 'Why can't I cry even though I'm sad?',
   verywell Mind, 12 August 2023, available at: www.verywellmind.
   com/reasons-why-you-aren-t-crying-5324069 (accessed August
   2024).

5. Read yourself sexy

1 Shirley Conran, *Lace* (Edinburgh: Canongate, 2012).
2 Sophie Kinsella, You're Booked Archive All-Stars, Season 14,
   Episode 160, 1 April 2024, available at: https://shows.acast.
   com/booked/episodes/sophie-kinsella (accessed August 2024).
3 Isy Suttie, You're Booked, Season 10, Episode 95, 9 August
   2021, available at: https://shows.acast.com/booked/episodes/
   isy-suttie (accessed August 2024).
4 Elizabeth Day, You're Booked Archive All-Stars, Season 14,
   Episode 158, 4 March 2024, available at: https://shows.acast.
   com/booked/episodes/elizabeth-day (accessed August 2024).
5 Halima Jibril, 'Why more and more young people are opting
   for voluntary celibacy', *Dazed*, 14 February 2023, available at:
   www.dazeddigital.com/life-culture/article/58185/1/young-
   people-choosing-voluntary-celibacy-gen-z-attitudes-sex-
   relationships (accessed August 2024).
6 Serena Smith, 'Rejoice! The sex recession is over', *Dazed*, 1
   March 2024, available at: www.dazeddigital.com/life-culture/
   article/62096/1/rejoice-the-sex-recession-is-over-gen-z-
   research (accessed August 2024).
7 Olivia Dean, 'Why socially inept Generation Z is having less
   sex than ever: They're over-therapised, underpaid, obsessed
   with social meda… and the dates are terrible', MailOnline,14
   March 2024, available at: www.dailymail.co.uk/femail/
   article-13193707/With-half-Gen-Z-living-home-scrolling-social-
   media-therapised-underpaid-despairing-OLIVIA-DEAN-asks-
   wonder-generation-having-no-sex.html   (accessed   August
   2024).

8   Clinical team, 'Is screen time damaging your sex life?', Lloyds Pharmacy Online Doctor, 24 April 2023, available at: https://onlinedoctor.lloydspharmacy.com/uk/sexual-health-advice/sex-and-screen-time#:~:text=1%20in%208%20women%20say,partner%20after%20looking%20at%20influencers (accessed August 2024).

9   Ellen Scott, 'So, how's watching Love Island every night affecting your sex life?', *Metro*, 14 July 2018, available at: https://metro.co.uk/2018/07/14/watching-love-island-every-night-affecting-sex-life-7715753 (accessed August 2024).

10 Hannah Fry, 'A "failure to launch": Why young people are having less sex', *Los Angeles Times*, 3 August 2023, available at: www.latimes.com/california/story/2023-08-03/young-adults-less-sex-gen-z-millennials-generations-parents-grandparents (accessed August 2024).

11 Annie Lord, 'What has growing up watching porn done to my brain – and my sex life', *The Guardian*, 12 February 2022, available at: www.theguardian.com/society/2022/feb/12/what-growing-up-watching-porn-has-done-to-my-brain-and-sex-life (accessed August 2024).

12 Zoe Cormier, 'Is porn bad for you?', BBC Science Focus, 8 May 2023, available at: www.sciencefocus.com/the-human-body/is-pornography-harmful (accessed August 2024).

13 Margaret Davis, 'Access to violent porn linked to rise in sexual crimes committed by children', *The Independent*, 10 January 2024, available at: www.independent.co.uk/news/uk/national-crime-agency-metropolitan-police-england-wales-data-b2476032.html (accessed August 2024).

14 'Mia Khalifa: Porn contracts "prey on vulnerable girls"', BBC News, 13 August 2019, available at: www.bbc.co.uk/news/newsbeat-49330540 (accessed August 2024).

15 Gwen Aviles, '*Fifty Shades of Grey* was the best-selling book of the decade', NBC News, 20 December 2019, available at: www.nbcnews.com/pop-culture/books/fifty-shades-grey-was-best-

selling-book-decade-n1105731 (accessed August 2024).

16 Brandie Welkie, 'Young female readers, #BookTok fuel spicy romantasy genre's staggering sales figures', CBC Radio, 25 February 2024, available at: www.cbc.ca/radio/day6/romantasy-booktok-female-readers-1.7120386 (accessed August 2024).

6. Reading your relatives

1 Leo Tolstoy, *Anna Karenina* (first published by T.Ris, Moscow, 1878; translated by Constance Garnett, London: William Heinemann, 1901; translated by Richard Pevear and Larissa Volokhonsky, London: Penguin, 2006).

2 Ram Dass, 'Ram Dass quotes', Ram Dass, n.d., available at: www.ramdass.org/ram-dass-quotes/?gad_source=1&gclid=CjwKCAjw5Ky1BhAgEiwA5jGujqnsVE6US9M1YQLb16SnwY75ValIvaQ1FpAjPEiKZ20N2V4lbCW36RoChGEQAvD_BwE (accessed August 2024).

3 Nancy Pearl, *Book Lust: Recommended reading for every mood, moment, and reason* (Seattle, WA: Sasquatch Books, 2003).

4 Anna North, 'You can't even pay people to have more kids', Vox, 27 November 2023, available at: www.vox.com/23971366/declining-birth-rate-fertility-babies-children (accessed August 2024).

5 Heather Stewart, 'Birthrate in UK falls to record low as campaigners say "procreation a luxury"', *The Guardian*, 23 February 2024, available at: www.theguardian.com/uk-news/2024/feb/23/birthrate-in-uk-falls-to-record-low-as-campaigners-say-procreation-is-a-luxury#:~:text=In%20total%2C%20there%20were%20605%2C479,recent%20years%2C%20including%20central%20London (accessed August 2024).

6 Sheila Heti, *Motherhood* (London: Vintage, 2019).

7. Read yourself free

1 Marian Keyes, *Rachel's Holiday* (London: Penguin, 1998).

2   Pema Chödrön, *When Things Fall Apart: Heart advice for difficult times* (Boulder, CO: Shambhala, 1996).

3   Keyes, *Rachel's Holiday*.

4   Keyes, *Rachel's Holiday*.

5   Emma Barnett, 'With ecstasy coming back, we need more campaigners like Leah Betts's parents', *The Guardian*, 26 January 2017, available at: www.theguardian.com/commentisfree/2017/jan/26/ecsasy-comeback-brave-parents-leah-betts-drugs (accessed August 2024).

6   Neil Strauss, 'Kurt Cobain's downward spiral: The last days of Nirvana's leader', *RollingStone*, 2 June 1994, available at: www.rollingstone.com/music/music-news/kurt-cobains-downward-spiral-the-last-days-of-nirvanas-leader-99797 (accessed August 2024).

7   Keyes, *Rachel's Holiday*.

8   Johann Hari, 'Johann Hari: "The opposite of addiction isn't sobriety – it's connection"', *The Guardian*, 21 April 2016, available at: www.theguardian.com/books/2016/apr/12/johann-hari-chasing-the-scream-war-on-drugs (accessed August 2024).

9   Sophie Kinsella, *The Secret Dreamworld of a Shopaholic* (London: Black Swan, 2000).

10 Laura McKowen, *We Are the Luckiest: The surprising magic of a sober life* (Novato, CA: New World Library, 2020).

11 McKowen, *We Are the Luckiest*.

12 Holly Whitaker, *Quit Like a Woman: The radical choice to not drink in a culture obsessed with alcohol* (London: Bloomsbury, 2020).

13 Whitaker, *Quit Like a Woman*.

14 Bryony Gordon, *Glorious Rock Bottom* (London: Headline, 2020).

15 Jilly Cooper, *Octavia* (London: Corgi, 1977).

16 Kenneth Grahame, *The Wind in the Willows* (first published, London: Methuen, 1908; London: Egmont, 2021).

8. Read yourself romantic

1 Dodie Smith, *I Capture the Castle* (first published, London: William Heinemann, 1949; London: Vintage, 2004).

2 John Waters, *Role Models* (London: Corsair, 2014).

3 'Your brain on books', Wellness@Mather, Mather Hospital, Northwell Health, n.d., available at: www.matherhospital.org/wellness-at-mather/diseases-conditions/your-brain-on-books (accessed August 2024).

4 Fred Cherrygarden, 'Istanbul 2461, Istanbul Museum of the Ancient Orient, Istanbul, Turkey: Quite possibly the oldest love poem known to humankind', Atlas Obscura, 18 March 2020, available at: www.atlasobscura.com/places/istanbul-2461 (accessed August 2024).

5 Will Dahlgreen, 'Shakespeare 400 years on: Every play ranked by popularity', YouGov UK, 22 April 2016, available at: https://yougov.co.uk/society/articles/15220-shakespeare-400 (accessed August 2024).

6 Gail Kern Paster, 'A modern perspective: Romeo and Juliet', Folger Shakespeare Library, n.d., available at: www.folger.edu/explore/shakespeares-works/romeo-and-juliet/romeo-and-juliet-a-modern-perspective (accessed August 2024).

7 'Sales of romance novels are rising in Britain', *The Economist*, 6 May 2023, available at: www.economist.com/britain/2023/03/06/sales-of-romance-novels-are-rising-in-britain (accessed August 2024).

8 Sinead Butler, 'Gen Z daters are scared of rejection and being cringe, according to Hinge', indy100, 11 February 2024, available at: www.indy100.com/lifestyle/gen-z-dating-habits-hinge (accessed August 2024).

9 Deanna Schwartz and Meghan Collins Sullivan, 'Gen Z is driving sales of romance books to the top of bestseller lists', NPR, 29 August 2022, available at: www.npr.org/2022/08/29/1119886246/gen-z-is-driving-sales-of-romance-books-to-the-top-of-bestseller-lists (accessed August 2024).

10 Nichi Hodgson, 'Young Brits say they are having less sex: Maybe that's not such a bad thing', *The Guardian*, 8 May 2019, available at: www.theguardian.com/commentisfree/2019/may/08/young-brits-less-sex-emotion-honest (accessed August 2024).

11 Nancy Mitford, *The Pursuit of Love and Other Novels* (The Pursuit of Love first published, London: Hamish Hamilton, 1945; London: Penguin, 2021).

12 'Divorce since 1900', UK Parliament, n.d. available at: www.parliament.uk/business/publications/research/olympic-britain/housing-and-home-life/split-pairs (accessed August 2024).

13 Having avoided the glamour and chaos of Linda's lifestyle in Mitford's first book, Fanny finds it later in Mitford's final novel, *Don't Tell Alfred* (first published, London: Hamish Hamilton, 1960; London: Penguin, 2015), in which Alfred is appointed the British Ambassador to France, and Fanny is uprooted to Paris.

14 Calhoun, Ada, *Wedding Toasts I'll Never Give* (New York: W. W. Norton & Company, 2018).

9. Reading like a writer

1 James B. Meriwether and Michael Millgate (eds), 'Year: 1947, Interview: Classroom Statements at the University of Mississippi', *Lion in the Garden: Interviews with William Faulkner 1926–1962* (Lincoln, NE: University of Nebraska Press, 1980).

2 Julie Cohen, You're Booked, Season 3, Episode 24, 13 May 2019, available at: https://shows.acast.com/booked/episodes/24.juliecohen (accessed August 2024).

3 National Geographic Society, 'Storytelling', *National Geographic*, 10 October 2023, available at: https://education.nationalgeographic.org/resource/storytelling-x (accessed August 2024).

4 James Norquay, 'How many emails are sent per day in 2024', Prosperity Media, 20 December 2024, available at: https://prosperitymedia.com.au/how-many-emails-are-sent-per-day-in-2024 (accessed August 2024).

5 Chantelle Pattemore, 'All about email anxiety', PsychCentral, 18

October 2022, available at: https://psychcentral.com/anxiety/email-anxiety#why-emails-anxiety (accessed August 2024).

6 Elizabeth Gilbert, *Big Magic: Creative living beyond fear* (London: Bloomsbury, 2015).

7 Anne Lamott, *Bird by Bird: Some instructions on writing and life* (Edinburgh: Canongate, 2020).

8 Lamott, *Bird by Bird*.

9 Oliver Burkeman, *Four Thousand Weeks: Time and how to use it* (London: The Bodley Head, 2021).

10. Reading beyond your comfort zone (and returning to it)

1 George Eliot, *Middlemarch* (first published, London and Edinburgh: William Blackwood & Sons, 1871–72; Oxford: Oxford University Press, 2019).

2 Nancy Pearl, *Book Lust: Recommended reading for every mood, moment, and reason* (Seattle, WA: Sasquatch Books, 2003).

3 Sarah Shaffi, 'Why we need to stop forcing ourselves to finish books we hate', *Stylist*, 2018, available at: www.stylist.co.uk/books/unfinished-books-should-you-stop-reading-books-dont-enjoy-guilt/279124 (accessed August 2024).

4 Nicholas Blincoe, 'Dickens muddled his racist caricatures', *The Guardian*, 17 December 2007, available at: www.theguardian.com/books/booksblog/2007/dec/17 dickensmuddledhisracistcar (accessed August 2024).

5 'Letters reveal Charles Dickens tried to place his wife in an asylum', University of York, 20 February 2019, available at: www.york.ac.uk/news-and-events/news/2019/research/dickens-letters-asylum/#:~:text=Cook%20writes%3A%20 'He%20discovered%20at,wrest%20it%20to%20his%20purpose (accessed August 2024).

6 Keyes' acclaimed novels have covered subjects including mental illness and addiction, and she was part of the successful 'Repeal' campaign, legalising abortion in Ireland. Her novel

The Break (London: Michael Joseph, 2017) features an Irish character travelling to England to terminate a pregnancy. See Anna Burnside, 'Irish author Marian Keyes reveals people burned her books because she supported repealing the Eighth Amendment', *Irish Mirror*, 30 May 2018, available at: www.irishmirror.ie/showbiz/irish-showbiz/irish-author-marian-keyes-reveals-12619821 (accessed August 2024).

7 Eliot, *Middlemarch*.

8 Katherine Woodfine, 'Why does my son re-read the same books', BookTrust, 30 October 2015, available at: www.booktrust.org.uk/news-and-features/features/2013/ask-book-trust---why-does-my-son-re-read-the-same-books   (accessed August 2024).

9 'Play for adults', National Institute for Play (NIFPlay), n.d., available at: www.nifplay.org/play-for-you/make-play-part-of-an-adult-life (accessed August 2024).

10 Brené Brown, 'The very best resolution you can make this year', Oprah.com, 2022, available at: www.oprah.com/omagazine/best-resolution-have-a-happy-year#:~:text=Brown%20believes%20that%20play%20is,to%20restrict%20play%20to%20vacations (accessed August 2024).

11 Brown, 'The very best resolution you can make this year'.

11. Reading for courage

1 Emma Donoghue, *Room* (London: Picador, 2010).

2 Malala Yousafzai, '16th birthday speech at the United Nations', Malala Fund, 12 July 2013, available at: https://malala.org/newsroom/malala-un-speech (accessed August 2024).

3 Amelia Tait, 'Greta Thunberg: How one teenager became the voice of the planet', *WIRED*, 6 June 2019, available at: www.wired.com/story/greta-thunberg-climate-crisis (accessed August 2024).

4 NoCamels Team, 'Age dramatically increases our fear of everything, study reveals', NoCamels, 4 June 2015, available at:

https://nocamels.com/2015/06/age-influences-perception-of-fear (accessed August 2024).

5 'Judith Kerr: A portrait of a fascinating life', BookTrust, 1 April 2010, available at: https://web.archive.org/web/20131203024744/http://www.booktrust.org.uk/books/children/illustrators/interviews/104 (accessed August 2024).

12. Reading around the world

1 Jean Rhys, *Wide Sargasso Sea* (first published, London: André Deutsch, 1966; London: Penguin, 2000).

2 'Definitions', in report '2020: Words of an unprecedented year', Oxford Languages, p. 32, available at: https://languages.oup.com/word-of-the-year/2020 (accessed August 2024).

3 Sophie Bushwick, 'How to stop doomscrolling news and social media', *Scientific American*, 12 February 2021, available at: www.scientificamerican.com/article/how-to-stop-doomscrolling-news-and-social-media (accessed August 2024).

4 Bonnie Evie Gifford, 'What is mean world syndrome?', Happiful, 18 September 2020, available at: https://happiful.com/what-is-mean-world-syndrome (accessed August 2024).

5 Alison Flood, 'Book sales surge as self-isolating readers top up on "bucket list" novels', *The Guardian*, 25 March 2020, available at: www.theguardian.com/books/2020/mar/25/book-sales-surge-self-isolating-readers-bucket-list-novels (accessed August 2024).

6 Kim Wilsher, 'Albert Camus' novel *The Plague* leads surge of pestilence fiction', *The Guardian*, 28 March 2020, available at: www.theguardian.com/books/2020/mar/28/albert-camus-novel-the-plague-la-peste-pestilence-fiction-coronavirus-lockdown (accessed August 2024).

7 Albert Camus, *The Plague*, translated by Laura Marris (New York: Vintage, 2022).

8 Adam Buxton, You're Booked, Season 15, Episode 168, 8 July 2024, available at: https://shows.acast.com/booked/episodes/adam-buxton (accessed August 2024).

9   Josie Long, You're Booked, Season 13, Episode 136, 5 June 2023, available at: https://shows.acast.com/booked/episodes/josie-long (accessed August 2024).
10 Emma Dabiri, You're Booked, Season 14, Episode 148, 16 October 2023, available at: https://shows.acast.com/booked/episodes/emma-dabiri (accessed August 2024).

Epilogue: Turning the page

1   Elif Shafak, *The Bastard of Istanbul* (London: Viking, 2007).

Bibliography

Introduction

Buchanan, Daisy, *Insatiable* (London: Sphere, 2022).

Buchanan, Daisy, *Careering* (London: Sphere, 2023).

Buchanan, Daisy, *Limelight* (London: Sphere, 2024).

Buchanan, Daisy, *Pity Party* (London: Sphere, 2025).

Green, John, *The Fault in Our Stars* (London: Penguin, 2013).

Smith, Ali, *How to Be Both* (London: Penguin, 2015).

1. Read yourself calmer

Angelou, Maya, *Life Doesn't Frighten Me*, edited by Sara Jane Boyers, illustrated by Jean Michel-Basquiat (New York: Abrams Books, 2018).

Caddy, Becca, *Screen Time: How to make peace with your devices and find your techquilibrium* (London: Blink, 2021).

Dobelli, Rolf, *The Art of Thinking Clearly: The secrets of perfect decision-making* (London: Sceptre, 2014).

Howard, Elizabeth Jane, Cazalet Chronicle Collection – *The Light Years; Marking Time; Confusion; Casting Off; All Change* (London: Pan, 2017).

Kolk, Bessel van der, *The Body Keeps the Score: Mind, brain and body in the transformation of trauma* (London: Penguin, 2015).

Lamott, Anne *Almost Everything: Notes on hope* (Edinburgh: Canongate, 2019).

Mort, Dr Sophie, *A Manual for Being Human: Practical advice for a happier life* (London: Simon & Schuster, 2022).

Williamson, Henry, *Tarka the Otter: His joyful water-life and death in the country of the two rivers* (first published, London and New York: G. P. Putnam's Sons, 1927; London: Puffin, 2014).

2. Read yourself secure

Austen, Jane, *Pride and Prejudice* (first published, London: T. Egerton, 1813; London: Penguin, 2003).

Dahl, Roald, *Matilda*, illustrated by Quentin Blake (London: Puffin, 2022).

Delafield, E. M., *Diary of a Provincial Lady* (first published, London: Macmillan, 1930; Pan Macmillan, 2016).

Digby, Anne, The Trebizon Boarding School 6 Books Collection Set (titles shortened) – *Second Term; Summer Term; Boy Trouble; More Trouble; Summer Camp; Tennis Term* (London: Egmont, 2020).

Fielding, Helen, *Bridget Jones's Diary* (London: Picador, 2014).

Grossmith, George and Weedon, *The Diary of a Nobody* (originally appeared in Punch, first published, Bristol: J. W. Arrowsmith, and London: Simpkin, Marshall, Hamilton , Kent & Co., 1892; London: Pan Macmillan, 2019).

Irby, Samantha, *Wow, No Thank You: Essays* (London: Faber & Faber, 2020).

Kuang, Rebecca F., *Yellowface* (London: The Borough Press, 2023).

Lehmann, Rosamond, *Invitation to the Waltz* (first published, London: Chatto & Windus, 1932; London: Virago, 2006).

May, Katherine, *Wintering: The power of rest and retreat in difficult times* (London: Rider, 2020).

Smith, Dodie, *I Capture the Castle* (first published, London: William Heinemann, 1949; London: Vintage, 2004).

Streatfeild, Noel, Gemma series – *Gemma Gemma and Sisters; Gemma Alone; and Good-bye Gemma* (London: HarperCollins, 1999).

Townsend, Sue, *The Secret Diary of Adrian Mole Aged 13¾* (London: Penguin, 2012).

Winn, Alice, *In Memoriam* (London: Penguin, 2024).

3. Read yourself funnier

Adams, Douglas, The Complete Hitchhiker's Guide to the Galaxy – *So Long and Thanks for All the Fish; Life the Universe and Everything; Mostly Harmless; The Hitchhiker's Guide to the Galaxy; and The Restaurant at the End of the Universe* (London: Pan, 2020).

Amis, Kingsley, *Lucky Jim* (London: Penguin, 2012).

Baxendale, Leo, *Willie the Kid* (London: Duckworth, 1976).

Bently, Peter and Matsuoka, Mei, *The Great Dog Bottom Swap* (London: Andersen Press, 2010).

Chast, Roz, *Can't We Talk About Something More Pleasant?: A memoir* (New York: Bloomsbury, 2016).

Delafield, E. M., *Diary of a Provincial Lady* (first published, London: Macmillan, 1930; Pan Macmillan, 2016).

Eldin, Peter, *The Tricksters' Handbook*, illustrated by Roger Smith (London: Armada, 1980).

Everett, Percival, *The Trees* (London: Picador, 2012).

Gibbons, Stella, *Cold Comfort Farm* (first published, London: Penguin, 1938; London: Penguin, 2020).

Greer, Andrew Sean, *Less* (London: Abacus, 2018).

Grossmith, George and Weedon, *The Diary of a Nobody* (originally appeared in Punch, first published, Bristol: J. W. Arrowsmith, and London: Simpkin, Marshall, Hamilton, Kent & Co., 1892; London: Pan Macmillan, 2019).

Hunter, Norman, *The Incredible Adventures of Professor Branestawm* (London: Puffin, 2015).

Jerome, K. Jerome, *Three Men in a Boat* (first published, Bristol: J. W. Arrowsmith, and London: Simpkin, Marshall, Hamilton, Kent & Co., 1889; London: Penguin, 2004).

Lederer, Helen, *Not That I'm Bitter* (London: Mirror Books, 2024).

Milne, A. A., *Winnie-the-Pooh*, illustrated by E. H. Shephard (first published, London: Methuen, 1926; London: Egmont, 2016).

Morris, Joel, *Be Funny or Die: How comedy works and why it matters* (London: Unbound, 2024).

Newman, Catherine, *We All Want Impossible Things* (London: Penguin, 2023).

Parker, Dorothy, *The Collected Dorothy Parker* (London: Penguin, 2001).

Stibbe, Nina, *Love, Nina: Despatches from family life* (London: Penguin, 2017).

Travis, Falcon and King, Colin, *The Usborne Spy's Guidebook* (London: Usborne, 1978).

4. Read it and weep

Barker, Elspeth, *O Caledonia* (London: Weidenfeld & Nicholson, 2021).

Brown, Craig, *Ma'am, Darling: 99 Glimpses of Princess Margaret* (London: 4th Estate, 2018).

Cameron, Julia, *The Artist's Way: A course in discovering and recovering your creative self* (London: Pan, 1995).

Comyns, Barbara, *Our Spoons Came from Woolworths* (London: Virago, 2013).

Cooper, Jilly, *Tackle!* (London: Penguin, 2024).

Doyle, Glennon, *Untamed* (London: Vermilion, 2020).

Jones, Tayari, *An American Marriage* (London: Oneworld, 2019).

Richardson, Samuel, *Pamela: or, Virtue Rewarded* (first published, London: C. Rivington and J. Osborn, 1740; Oxford: Oxford University Press, 2008).

White, E. B., *Charlotte's Web*, illustrated by Garth Williams (first published, London: Hamish Hamilton, 1952; London: Puffin, 2014).

Yanagihara, Hanya, *A Little Life* (London: Picador, 2017).

Zevin, Gabrielle, *Tomorrow, and Tomorrow, and Tomorrow* (London: Vintage, 2023).

5. Read yourself sexy

Austen, Jane, *Emma* (first published, London: John Murray, 1815; London: Penguin, 2015).

Baker, Nicholson, *Vox* (London: Granta, 2011).

Baker, Nicholson, *House of Holes* (London: Simon & Schuster, 2012).

Blume, Judy, *Forever* (London: Macmillan, 2015).

Buchanan, Daisy *Insatiable* (London: Sphere, 2022).

Caldwell, Lucy, *Intimacies* (London: Faber & Faber, 2021).

Collins, Jackie, *The Stud* (London: Simon & Schuster, 2021).

Conran, Shirley, *Lace* (Edinburgh: Canongate, 2012).

Cooper, Jilly, *Harriet* (London: Corgi, 2005).

Cooper, Jilly, *Rivals* (London: Corgi, 2007).

Cooper, Jilly, *Riders* (London: Corgi, 2015).

James, E. L., *Fifty Shades of Grey* (London: Century, 2012).

Jaswal, Balli Kaur, *Erotic Stories for Punjabi Widows* (London: HarperCollins, 2017).

Laclos, Choderlos de, *Les Liaisons Dangereuses*, translated and edited by Douglas Parmée (Oxford: Oxford University Press, 2008).

6. Reading your relatives

Alcott, Louisa May, *Little Women* (first published, Boston, MA: Roberts Brothers, 1868; London: Penguin, 2018).

Austen, Jane, *Pride and Prejudice* (first published, London: T. Egerton, 1813; London: Penguin, 2003).

Colwin, Laurie, *Happy All the Time* (London: Weidenfeld & Nicholson, 2021).

Cusk, Rachel, *A Life's Work* (London: Faber & Faber, 2019).

Dahl, Roald, *James and the Giant Peach*, illustrated by Quentin Blake (London: Puffin, 2022).

Dahl, Roald, *Matilda*, illustrated by Quentin Blake (London: Puffin, 2022).

Frizzell, Nell, *The Panic Year: Dates, doubts and the mother of all decisions* (London: Penguin, 2022).

Gannon, Emma, *Olive* (London: HarperCollins, 2020).

Gilbert, Elizabeth, *Eat Pray Love: One woman's search for everything* (London: Bloomsbury, 2007).

Heti, Sheila, *Motherhood* (London: Vintage, 2019).

Howard, Elizabeth Jane, Cazalet Chronicle Collection – *The Light Years; Marking Time; Confusion; Casting Off; All Change* (London: Pan, 2017).

Jones, Lucy, *Matrescence: On the metamorphosis of pregnancy, childbirth and motherhood* (London: Penguin, 2024).

Keyes, Marian, *The Mystery of Mercy Close* (London: Penguin, 2013).

Kilroy, Claire, *Soldier Sailor* (London: Faber & Faber, 2024).
Maupin, Armistead, Tales of the City series – *28 Barbary Lane: Tales of the City Books 1–3; Back to Barbary Lane: Tales of the City Books 4–6; Barbary Lane: Tales of the City Books 7–9* (London: HarperCollins, 2016).

Mendelson, Charlotte, *The Exhibitionist* (London: Picador, 2023).

Mitford, Nancy, *The Pursuit of Love and Other Novels (The Pursuit of Love* first published, London: Hamish Hamilton, 1945; London: Penguin, 2021).

Pearl, Nancy, *Book Lust: Recommended reading for every mood, moment, and reason* (Seattle, WA: Sasquatch Books, 2003).

Rowling, J. K., Harry Potter: The Complete Collection (titles shortened) – *The Philosopher's Stone; The Chamber of Secrets; The Prisoner of Azkaban; The Goblet of Fire; The Order of the Phoenix; The Half-Blood Prince; The Deathly Hallows* (London: Bloomsbury, 2018).

Smith, Dodie, *I Capture the Castle* (first published, London: William Heinemann, 1949; London: Vintage, 2004).

Streatfcild, Noel, *Ballet Shoes* (first published, London: J. M. Dent, 1936; London: Picador, 2023).

Stroud, Clover, *My Wild and Sleepless Nights: A mother's story* (London: Doubleday, 2021).

Sukumar, Hema, *Minor Disturbances at Grand Life Apartments* (London: Coronet, 2024).

Tolstoy, Leo, *Anna Karenina* (first published by T.Ris, Moscow, 1878; translated by Constance Garnett, London: William

Heinemann, 1901; translated by Richard Pevear and Larissa Volokhonsky, London: Penguin, 2006).

Trapido, Barbara, *Brother of the More Famous Jack* (London: Bloomsbury, 2022).

Whipple, Dorothy, *Someone at a Distance* (London: John Murray, 1953; London: Persephone Books, 2011).

Wilson, Jacqueline, *The Suitcase Kid*, illustrated by Nick Sharratt (London: Corgi Yearling, 2006).

Wilson, Jacqueline, *The Illustrated Mum*, illustrated by Nick Sharratt (London: Corgi Yearling, 2012).

Wilson, Jacqueline, *Girls in Love*, illustrated by Nick Sharratt (London: Corgi, 2016).

7. Read yourself free

Blyton, Enid, Malory Towers: The 12 Books Complete Collection (titles shortened) – *First Term; Second Term; Third Year; Upper Fourth; In the Fifth; Last Term; New Term; Summer Term; Winter Term; Fun and Games; Secrets; Goodbye* (London: Hodder & Stoughton, 2020).

Burgess, Melvyn, *Junk* (London: Andersen Press, 2020).

Burroughs, Augusten, *Dry: A memoir* (London: Atlantic Books, 2005).

Chödrön, Pema, *When Things Fall Apart: Heart advice for difficult times* (Boulder, CO: Shambhala, 1996).

Coffield, Darren, *Tales from the Colony Room: Soho's lost bohemia* (London: Unbound, 2021).

Cooper, Jilly, *Octavia* (London: Corgi, 1977).

Fielding, Helen, *Bridget Jones's Diary* (London: Picador, 2014).
Gordon, Bryony, *Glorious Rock Bottom* (London: Headline, 2020).

Grahame, Kenneth, *The Wind in the Willows* (first published, London: Methuen, 1908; London: Egmont, 2021).

Gray, Catherine, *The Unexpected Joy of Being Sober* (London: Aster, 2017).

Gray, Catherine, *The Unexpected Joy of the Ordinary* (London: Aster, 2023).

Keyes, Marian, *Rachel's Holiday* (London: Penguin, 1998).

Kinsella, Sophie, *The Secret Dreamworld of a Shopaholic* (London: Black Swan, 2000).

McKowen, Laura, *We Are the Luckiest: The surprising magic of a sober life* (Novato, CA: New World Library, 2020).

Welsh, Irvine, *Trainspotting* (London: Vintage, 1994).

Whitaker, Holly, *Quit Like a Woman: The radical choice to not drink in a culture obsessed with alcohol* (London: Bloomsbury, 2020).

8. Read yourself romantic

Alderton, Dolly, *Everything I Know About Love* (London: Penguin, 2024).

Ames, Jonathan, *I Love You More Than You Know* (New York: Black Cat, 2005).
Austen, Jane, *Pride and Prejudice* (first published, London: T. Egerton, 1813; London: Penguin, 2003).

Austen, Jane, *Emma* (first published, London: John Murray, 1815; London: Penguin, 2015).

Brontë, Charlotte, *Jane Eyre* (first published, London: Smith, Elder & Co., 1847; London: Penguin, 2006).

Calhoun, Ada, *Wedding Toasts I'll Never Give* (New York: W. W. Norton & Company, 2018).

Dickens, Charles, *Great Expectations* (first published, London: Chapman & Hall, 1861; Glasgow: William Collins, 2010).

Fitzgerald, F. Scott, *The Great Gatsby* (first published, New York: Charles Scribner's Sons, 1925; London: Penguin, 2000).

Fitzgerald, F. Scott, *Tender Is the Night* (first published, New York: Charles Scribner's Sons, 1934; Glasgow: William Collins, 2018).

Hardy, Thomas, *Far from the Madding Crowd* (first published, London: Smith, Elder & Co., 1874; Glasgow: William Collins, 2010).

Hardy, Thomas, *Tess of the D'Urbervilles* (first published, London: James R. Osgood, McIlvaine & Co., 1891; Glasgow: William Collins, 2010).

Heiny, Katherine, *Early Morning Riser* (London: 4th Estate, 2022).

Keane, Molly, *Good Behaviour* (London: Virago, 2005).

Keyes, Marian, *My Favourite Mistake* (London: Penguin, 2025).
Mitford, Nancy, *The Pursuit of Love and Other Novels* (The Pursuit of Love first published, London: Hamish Hamilton, 1945; London: Penguin, 2021).

Mitford, Nancy, *Don't Tell Alfred* (London: Hamish Hamilton, 1960; London: Penguin, 2015).

Nicholls, David, *Us* (London: Sceptre, 2015).

Nicholls, David, *One Day* (London: Hodder, 2024).

Nicholls, David, *You Are Here* (London: Sceptre, 2024).

O'Leary, Beth, *The Flatshare* (London: Quercus, 2022).

Pasternack, Boris, *Dr Zhivago*, translated by Max Hayward and Manya Harari (London: Vintage, 2002).

Salter, James, *Light Years* (London: Penguin, 2007).

Shakespeare, *Romeo and Juliet: The New Oxford Shakespeare* (first published, London: printed by John Danter and Edward Alide, 1597; Oxford: Oxford University Press, 2024).

Shields, Carol, *Larry's Party* (London: 4th Estate, 2010).

Smith, Dodie, *I Capture the Castle* (first published, London: William Heinemann, 1949; London: Vintage, 2004).

John Waters, *Role Models* (London: Corsair, 2014).

Wodehouse, P. G., *The Indiscretions of Archie* (Zinc Read, 2023).

9. Reading like a writer

Burkeman, Oliver, *Four Thousand Weeks: Time and how to use it* (London: The Bodley Head, 2021).

Gilbert, Elizabeth, *Big Magic: Creative living beyond fear* (London: Bloomsbury, 2015).

King, Stephen, *On Writing: a memoir of the craft* (London: Hodder & Stoughton, 2012).

Lamott, Anne, *Bird by Bird: Some instructions on writing and life* (Edinburgh: Canongate, 2020).

Robertson, Robin (ed.), *Mortification: Writers' stories of their public shame* (London: Harper, 2005).

Shukla, Nikesh, *Your Story Matters: Sharpen your writing skills, find your voice, tell your story* (London: Bluebird , 2023).

10. Reading beyond your comfort zone (and returning to it)

Blyton, Enid, *In the Fifth at Malory Towers* (London: Hodder & Stoughton, 2016).

Blyton, Enid, *The Magic Faraway Tree Collection* (London: Hodder & Stoughton, 2020).

Cleary, Beverly, *Beezus and Ramona*, illustrated by Jacqueline Rogers (London: HarperCollins, 2022).

Collins, Suzanne, *The Hunger Games* (London: Scholastic, 2011).

Cooper, Jilly, *Rivals* (London: Corgi, 2007).

Dickens, Charles, *A Christmas Carol* (first published, London: Chapman & Hall, 1843; London: Harper, 2013).

Dickens, Charles, *Great Expectations* (first published, London: Chapman & Hall, 1861; Glasgow: William Collins, 2010).

Dyer, Geoff, *The Colour of Memory* (Edinburgh: Canongate, 2012).

Eliot, George, *Middlemarch* (first published, London and Edinburgh: William Blackwood & Sons, 1871–72; Oxford: Oxford University Press, 2019).

Fisher, Carrie, *Postcards from the Edge* (London, Simon & Schuster, 2011).

Garnett, Eve, *The Family from One End Street* (London: Puffin, 2014).

Jewell, Lisa, *Ralph's Party* (London: Penguin, 2024).

Keyes, Marian, *The Break* (London: Michael Joseph, 2017).

Kinsella, Sophie, Shopaholic books (all published, London: Black Swan) – *The Secret Dreamworld of a Shopaholic* (2012); *Shopaholic Abroad* (2012); *Shopaholic Ties the Knot* (2012); *Shopaholic and Sister* (2005); *Shopaholic and Baby* (2007); *Mini Shopaholic* (2011); *Shopaholic to the Stars* (2015); *Shopaholic to the Rescue* (2016); *Christmas Shopaholic* (2020).

Mailer, Norman, *The Naked and the Dead* (London: Penguin, 2018).

Pearl, Nancy, *Book Lust: Recommended reading for every mood, moment, and reason* (Seattle, WA: Sasquatch Books, 2003).

Rowling, J. K., Harry Potter: The Complete Collection – see under Chapter 6.
Sittenfeld, Curtis, *American Wife* (London: Black Swan, 2009).

Streatfeild, Noel, *Ballet Shoes* (first published, London: J. M. Dent, 1936; London: Picador, 2023).

Walker, Fiona, *French Relations* (London: Coronet, 2004).

11. Reading for courage

Blyton, Enid, The Famous Five Library, boxed set of all 21 books (London: Hodder, 2016).

Donoghue, Emma, *Room* (London: Picador, 2022).

Ellman, Lucy, *Ducks, Newburyport* (Norwich, Norfolk: Galley Beggar Press, 2019).

Evaristo, Bernadine, *Girl, Woman, Other* (London: Penguin, 2020).

Godfrey, Jennie, *The List of Suspicious Things* (London: Penguin, 2025).

Kerr, Judith, *When Hitler Stole Pink Rabbit* (London: HarperCollins, 2017).

Nzelu, Okechuckwu, *Here Again Now* (London: Dialogue Books, 2022).

Rowling, J. K., Harry Potter: The Complete Collection – see under Chapter 6.

Tolkien, J. R. R., *The Hobbit* and *The Lord of the Rings* Boxed Set (London: HarperCollins, 1997).

Woodall, Trinny, *Fearless* (London: HQ, 2023).

12. Reading around the world

Camus, Albert, *The Plague* (first published as *La Peste*, Paris: Gallimard, 1947; translated by Laura Marris, New York: Vintage, 2022).

Daré, Abi, *The Girl with the Louding Voice* (London: Sceptre, 2020).

Deleuze, Gilles and Guattari, Félix, *A Thousand Plateaus: Capitalism and schizophrenia*, translated and foreword by Brian Massumi (London: Bloomsbury, 2013).

Ferrante, Elena, *My Brilliant Friend*, translated by Ann Goldstein (London: Europa Editions, 2020).

Fielding, Helen, *Cause Celeb* (London: Penguin, 2002).

Gopnik, Adam, *A Thousand Small Sanities: The moral adventure of liberalism* (London: Riverrun, 2020).

Hopkins, Rob, *From What Is to What If: Unleashing the power of imagination to create the future we want* (London: Chelsea Green, 2021).

Lalwani, Nikita, *You People* (London: Penguin, 2021).

Morgan, Ann, *Reading the World: How I read a book from every country* (London: Vintage, 2022).

Rhys, Jean, *Wide Sargasso Sea* (first published, London: André Deutsch, 1966; London: Penguin, 2000).

Saad, Layla F., *Me and White Supremacy: How to recognise your privilege, combat racism and change the world* (London: Quercus, 2022).

Toews, Miriam, *Women Talking: A novel* (London: Bloomsbury, 2018).

Wynne, Frank, *Found in Translation: 100 of the finest short stories ever translated* (London: Apollo, 2018).

Epilogue: Turning the page

Dolby, Hannah, *How to Solve Murders Like a Lady* (London: Head of Zeus, 2024).

Shafak, Elif, *The Bastard of Istanbul* (London: Viking, 2007).

Morgan, Ann, *Reading the World: How I read a book from every country* (London: Vintage, 2022).

Books that bring joy

Adams, Douglas and Lloyd, John, *The Meaning of Liff: The original dictionary of things there should be words for* (London: Faber & Faber and Boxtree, 2013).

Austen, Jane, *Persuasion* (first published, London: John Murray, 1818; London: Penguin, 2012).

Baker, Sam, *The Shift: How I lost and found myself after 40 – and you can too* (London: Coronet, 2021).

Bravo, Lauren, *Probably Nothing* (London: Simon & Schuster, 2025).

Brown, Kat (ed.), *No One Talks About This Stuff: Twenty-two stories of almost parenthood* (London: Unbound, 2024).

Collodi, Carlo, *The Adventures of Pinocchio: Story of a puppet*, translated by John Hooper and Ann Kraczyna (London: Penguin, 2021).

Colwin, Laurie, *Happy All the Time* (London: Weidenfeld & Nicholson, 2021).

Connelly, Charlie, *Attention All Shipping: A journey around the shipping forecast* (London: Abacus, 2005).

Cotton, Fearne, *Scripted* (London: Penguin Michael Joseph, 2024).

Crompton, Richmal, Just William Boxed Set: First 10 books – *Just William; More William; William Again; William the Fourth; Still William; William the Conqueror; William the Outlaw; William in Trouble; William the Good; William at War* (London: Macmillan, 1999).

Dickson Wright, Clarissa, *Spilling the Beans* (London: Hodder & Stoughton, 2008).

Fielding, Helen, *Bridget Jones: The edge of reason* (London: Picador, 2018).

Frizzell, Nell, *Cuckoo* (London: Penguin, 2025).

Gibbons, Stella, *Cold Comfort Farm* (first published, London: Penguin, 1938; London: Penguin, 2020).

Godfrey, Jennie, *The List of Suspicious Things* (London: Penguin, 2025).

Heiny, Katherine, *Standard Deviation* (London: 4th Estate, 2018).

Hession, Rónán, *Leonard and Hungry Paul* (Hebden Bridge, West Yorkshire: Bluemoose Books, 2019).

Honeyman, Gail, *Eleanor Oliphant is Completely Fine* (London: HarperCollins, 2018).

Hunter Murray, Andrew, *A Beginners' Guide to Breaking and Entering* (London: Hutchinson Heinemann, 2024).

Ince, Robin, *Bibliomaniac: An obsessive's tour of the bookshops of Britain* (London: Atlantic Books, 2022).

Keegan, Claire, *Foster* (London: Faber & Faber, 2022).

Keyes, Marian, *My Favourite Mistake* (London: Penguin, 2025).

Mackintosh, Clare, *I Let You Go* (London: Sphere, 2015).

Mandel, Emily St. John, *Station Eleven* (London: Picador, 2015).

Mason, Meg, *Sorrow and Bliss* (London: Weidenfeld & Nicholson, 2022).

May, Katherine, *Wintering: The power of rest and retreat in difficult times* (London: Rider, 2020).

May, Nikki, *This Motherless Land* (London: Penguin, 2025).

Mitford, Nancy, *The Pursuit of Love and Other Novels* (*The Pursuit of Love* first published, London: Hamish Hamilton, 1945; London: Penguin, 2021).

Moriarty, Jaclyn, *Gravity is the Thing* (London: Allen & Unwin, 2020).

Nicholls, David, *You Are Here* (London: Sceptre, 2025).

O'Brien, Edna, *The Country Girls,* in The Country Girls Trilogy: *The Country Girls, The Lonely Girl,* and *Girls in Their Married Bliss* (London: Faber & Faber, 2019).

Rentzenbrink, Cathy, *How to Feel Better: A guide to navigating the ebb and flow of life* (London: Bluebird, 2023).

Ruiz, Don Miguel, with Mills, Janet, *The Four Agreements: A practical guide to personal freedom* (San Rafael, CA: Amber-Allen Publishing, 2018).

Salinger, J. D., *Franny and Zooey* (London: Penguin, 2010).

Shaw, Dale, *Painfully British Haikus* (London: Penguin, 2019).

Shields, Carol, *Larry's Party* (London: 4th Estate, 2010).

Smith, Dodie, *I Capture the Castle* (first published, London: William Heinemann, 1949; London: Vintage, 2004).

Stibbe, Nina, *Went to London, Took the Dog: The diary of a 60-year-old runaway* (London: Picador, 2024).

Strout, Elizabeth, *My Name is Lucy Barton: A novel* (London: Penguin, 2017).

Townsend Warner, Sylvia, *Lolly Willowes: or The Loving Huntsman* (first published, London: Chatto & Windus, 1926; London: Penguin, 2020).

Trapido, Barbara, *Brother of the More Famous Jack* (London: Bloomsbury, 2022).

Tyler, Anne, *The Accidental Tourist* (London: Vintage, 2016).

Waller, Ericka, *Goodbye Birdie Greenwing* (London: Penguin, 2025).

Watson, Winifred, *Miss Pettigrew Lives for a Day* (first published, London: Methuen, 1938; London: Persephone Books, 2011).

Williams, Holly, *The Start of Something* (London: Orion, 2025).

About the author

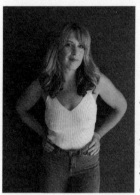

Sarah Kate Photography

Daisy Buchanan is an award-winning journalist, author, and broadcaster. She hosts the chart-topping podcast, You're Booked, where she interviews legendary writers from all over the world about their reading habits. She often appears on *Woman's Hour*, *Times Radio*, and *Good Morning Britain* and has written several novels including the bestselling *Insatiable* (Sphere, 2021) and *Careering* (Sphere, 2022) which was adapted by Radio Four and selected for the BBC Sounds Book Club.